STANDING UP!

My Story OF **HOPE, ADVOCACY** & **SURVIVAL** after Stroke

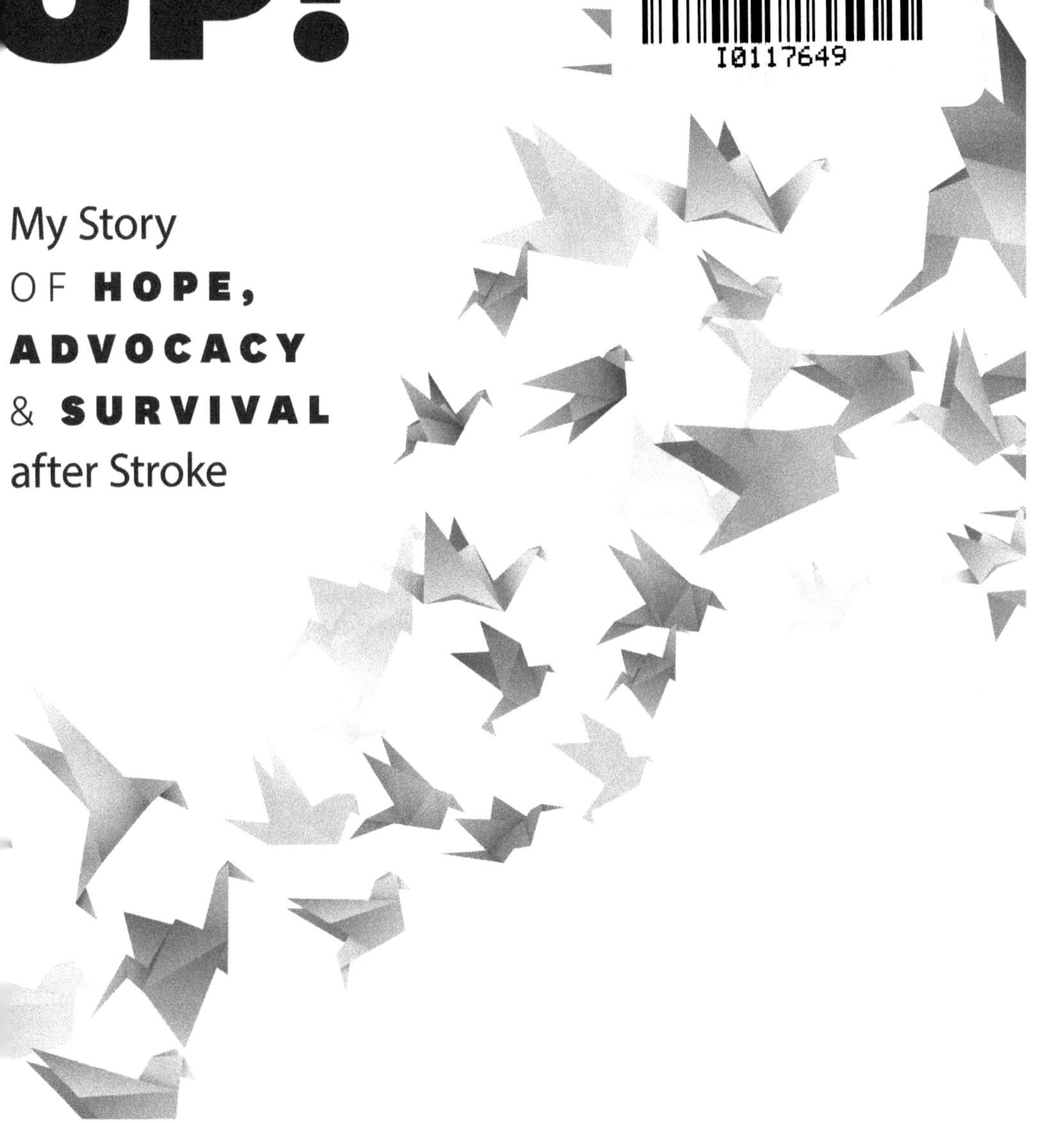

Kathleen Jordan

with Vicki Steggall

Standing Up: My Story of Hope, Advocacy and Survival after Stroke
by Kathleen Jordan

National Library of Australia cataloguing-in-publication data:
Author: Jordan, Kathleen
Memoir, self-help and personal development

ISBN 9780648460442 (pb)
ISBN 9780648460459 (ebk)

Cover image: Shutterstock

Design: Working Type Studio, Melbourne
Production: Jasmine Standfield

Praise for Standing Up!

In sharing her deeply personal experience of a severe stroke and road to recovery, Kathleen has given the reader an insight into the physical challenges faced by stroke victims and the emotional and mental challenges facing them and those who love them. The book is a masterclass in resilience and humanity.

Cecilia Burgess, COO of Bell Gully Lawyers NZ and former client

Kathleen is an extraordinary and inspirational human being. She is a shining example of what it takes to look adversity straight in the eye and have the courage to say 'go away, you certainly will not get the better of me... not ever!' Standing Up! *illustrates the extraordinary and harrowing physical and psychological ordeal Kathleen experienced, reflecting her remarkable determination, fortitude and passionate will to succeed.*

Her story is a compelling and inspirational one that will move you to appreciate and see your life and all that is in it in a new light. The book is beautifully and compassionately written. It will move you in a deep, profound and loving way!

Bernadette Baynie, Group General Counsel, Batelco Group

Kathleen Jordan inspired leaders to new heights before her stroke and now with this book she continues to inspire us with her story about how she dealt with what life threw at her. To have come through her stroke experience with such a strong desire to contribute what she learned to others is truly remarkable. Her practical approach to her recovery offers something for all of us as we deal with those curve balls that life throws at us.

Brian Donovan, Director, Donovan Leadership

Jordan's book vividly expresses the vital but multi layered complicated processes of standing up for herself (with the support of her Hope Team of family and friends) as she negotiated her way through bureaucracy and 'the system' following a catastrophic stroke.

After years of sadness and loss, unanswered questions and disappointing rehabilitation encounters, Jordan and her family continued to struggle, learn, and endeavour to put every effort into her regaining her feet so she could leave her wheelchair and stand up. Bravo!

Standing Up! *stands up for the importance of family, friends, kindness, purpose, love and hope to stand up to stroke.*

Dr Christine Durham, Victorian Senior Australian of the Year 2014, BrainLink Woman of Achievement 2012 and author of *Unlocking my Brain*, Ventura Press 2014

This is a true story of survival... a compelling story about the experience of and recovery from stroke — a massive assault on the brain's structure and functioning, and on life as it was. It is the sort of book from which any stroke sufferer could gain great support, encouragement, strength and courage. But it is much more than this. It is a story of family, of grief, of love, of despair, of determination, and of hope and belief... a story that will resonate with many others who have travelled a parallel journey.

The title Standing Up! *couldn't be more apt. The author gives a moving account of the sometimes agonising process of learning how to compensate for the breakdown in communication between her brain and her body, and of relearning what able-bodied people consider to be the most basic of physical actions. She also writes of the emotional 'standing up' that needed to happen, initially by family members on her behalf, and later by Kathleen herself, in relation to a medical and service provision system that required standing up to. The lessons learned here were crucial, and will potentially serve as an invaluable aid to families in the future.*

Kathleen's writing is a life-affirming, lively and loving account. Well before her stroke and the writing of this book, Kathleen expressed her goal for living her passion: 'Bringing love, generosity and inspiration to the world.'

Her stroke, far from preventing her from doing this, has enabled this particular manifestation of exactly that. May it inspire others to identify and nurture their own.

Pamela Rycroft, Psychologist and Family Therapist

Positive psychology is a key part of the Melbourne Graduate School of Education's approach to developing the teachers of the future. This emerging discipline is helping to prepare children and young people to live flourishing lives. In Standing Up! *Kathleen shows how positive psychology tools helped her back from the brink after a major stroke. I strongly recommend this book to anyone going through major life changes.*

Professor Field Rickards, Dean, Melbourne Graduate School of Education, University of Melbourne

This book is a powerful testament to both the isolating effects of injury to the brain — that you've got to find your own way to recovery and adaptation — and the crucial role that family and friends play in that journey. It is required reading for every clinician and allied health professional working with people who experience stroke.

Nick Rushworth, Executive Officer,
Brain Injury Australia

A crisis can be turned into a challenge, it all depends on how you choose to look at it. Kathleen has made choices she never considered possible or necessary. As I read her journey I felt shocked, saddened, amazed, humbled, grateful, lucky and at times I laughed out loud. Having spent time with Kathleen during those two years in rehab, I can now see and hear and feel the distance between where she was and where she is now. Strength of mind is desirable and at times elusive for us all and this is a personal account of many mountains which have already been climbed and those which are still being challenged. Favourite cousin, you are one hell of a woman!

Paula Day

Resilience is one of the pillars for today's business leaders. This book is a story of resilience that will move you and continue to teach long after you have reluctantly turned the last page.

Dr Megan Clark AC, Advisory Board member, Bank of America Merrill Lynch

Kathleen shares an honest and moving narrative of her experiences post brain injury. She faces fear, hopelessness and despair not only of the condition itself but of the care system which often failed her. Alongside her family and friends she holds onto hope and determination to live her *life* her *way. Her story will inspire individuals and their family members struggling with the aftermath of brain injury and provide insight to workers in their caring role.*

Franca Butera-Prinzi, Social Worker/ Family Therapist

I have known Kathleen for some time, both as a friend and as a valued and trusted adviser to our business.

Kathleen's story is one sometimes of despair, deep frustration and overwhelming loss, but also one of remarkable courage and dogged determination to recover from a debilitating illness, and the cruel and sudden loss of independence and all she held dear and had worked so hard to establish.

Her story is also a reminder to us all of the strength of family and close friends and how we need to nurture those relationships that so enrich us, but that we sometimes take so much for granted.

Kathleen's continuing bravery in the face of the profound loss of her daughter, Lucinda, is also both heart-rending and inspirational.

On behalf of myself and my colleagues at Cornwall Stodart, I wish Kathleen all the luck in the world in her efforts to return to full mobility.

Michelle McLean, Chief Executive Officer,
Cornwall Stodart, Melbourne

This is a wonderful book. I found it a compelling read. First I relived my dear friend Kathleen's horrific stroke and family tragedies and the ongoing story of her courageous and inspirational recovery. The book then took me to the strategies she drew upon to help her with her recovery — all of which she'd used with clients in her professional life. A must read for everyone in the stroke community — both those who've had a stroke and their families, and the clinical and research teams working in the field. And it's also a good read for anyone who enjoys a well told story about the power of the human spirit.

Kate Ramsay, AnD Leadership Consulting

This book is dedicated to my two daughters,
Emma and Lucinda, whose love and support
has been instrumental in my being alive today.

To Emma Patricia Keldan, my first born,
with eternal love and gratitude.

And in loving memory of Dr Lucinda May Jordan,
28 April 1978 to 5 May 2015.
A loving, sassy, intelligent and beautiful soul.

About the authors

Kathleen Jordan is a leadership and development coach working with major corporations, and across various levels of government, law firms and not for profit organisations. Kathleen launched her business, iNTUITIVE iNSIGHTS, in 1995 and has since travelled nationally and internationally working with high-level executives and their management teams. Kathleen was also a board member of the Bionic Ear Institute for 16 years. www.intuitivesights.com.au

Vicki Steggall has been writing professionally for over 25 years. Her work has appeared in numerous books, journals, magazines, and newspapers. In addition to co-authoring or writing non-fiction books she has published two best-selling children's books. Her most recently published works include *In Your Face,* a perspective on the history and effects of plastic surgery, and *Anything Can Happen,* the story of the early years of the iconic Australian fashion retailer, Sportsgirl. She is currently working on two memoirs and a series of children's books. www.vickisteggall.com.au

Preface

This story gives a compelling insight into the effects of a major stroke that strikes down a vibrant businesswoman, mother and grandmother and her amazing recovery.

Kathleen Jordan, with Vicki Steggall, recounts her stroke journey through the acute trauma, the stroke ward, short and long-term rehabilitation units and, finally, her return to semi-normalcy and everyday life.

There are numerous lessons for every reader in this accessible, emotional and raw story of triumph over adversity.

Standing Up! offers a unique and privileged view of the treating medical staff, the amazing nurses and allied health professionals and, above all, what an extended but close family and friendship network can do to rehabilitate their loved one.

Advocacy, determination and constant belief shine through.

The sheer tenacity of the patient in confronting and conquering the challenges of stroke requires an extraordinary sense of self-belief, founded on core values and working with professional advice.

As Kathleen is recovering, she shares with the reader her personal anguish at the loss of her parents and, tragically, her daughter to cancer.

The second part of this story provides a framework of the literature and resources available to support stroke survivors and their carers. Kathleen's international experience with leadership coaching and consulting bears directly on the techniques she offers, with simple, effective ideas and quotations that will stir your soul.

In closing, to have worked with Kathleen in her former capacity on the board of a major medical research unit and now to have followed her stroke journey is a unique privilege which reinforces the need for the community to know more about stroke, that is preventable, treatable and beatable.

Kathleen is a heroine and her story must be read.

Professor James Angus AO
President, National Stroke Foundation

This is the story of the stroke that I suffered on 23 August 2011 and, more particularly, of the months and years that followed. It is based on my memories and those of my family, who deputised for me in the early post-stroke months and whose extraordinary efforts undoubtedly changed the outcome for me.

There are always many viewpoints about how events unfold. I have been as accurate as I can, but this remains a personal story about my experience.

I have learnt so much from my recovery — about life, about the way our thoughts can help or hinder our progress, and on the need to be open to my new life. I hope what I learnt will help other patients and their families.

Kathleen Jordan

Prelude

I'm racing down Flemington Road in the back of an intensive care ambulance. Faces loom over me, kind questions are asked, but my brain keeps replaying the meeting I have just ruined by collapsing part way through. I'm annoyed to think that it's now receding into the distance behind me. My addled brain sees it in terms of distance and geography, but what's really happening is that, along with the rest of my life, it's receding into time. It's becoming another era and it will be years before I'm back.

I had a dizzy spell. There have been others, each dramatic but not serious. I'm 62, have moderately raised blood pressure, controlled by tablets and exercise, plus all the usual stresses. That fact that this meeting meant a lot to me no doubt triggered the dizziness. I had been presenting an idea at the Royal Children's Hospital to boost research into a rare neurological disorder called Angelman Syndrome, a syndrome affecting my grandson, so I was understandably anxious.

Instead, rather dramatically, I'm leaving as a potential neurological patient myself.

When the paramedic speaks kindly, gratitude for this stranger flows over me, calming my cycle of fear and aggravation. But when I look up he seems to have disappeared, along with the interior of the ambulance.

I've spent my life being independent, bringing up my daughters and creating a business that takes me around the world consulting to large corporations. I'm on the board of the

Bionic Ear Institute (now the Bionics Institute). I'm a mother, a grandmother and about to take on an activist role in an area of children's health.

And yet here I am, strapped to a trolley, swaying nauseatingly in an ambulance, being rushed to the emergency department. Someone's hand holds mine. From the Children's Hospital to the Royal Melbourne Hospital is only a kilometre, but it seems to be taking a lot longer.

Really, I don't have time for this.

23 August 2011

The day of the stroke — the start of the journey

There is so much to learn when you are uprooted from the everyday journey of life to the journey of survival from stroke. My first lesson arrived along with the first symptoms. It was about the power others have to give hope and respect, or destroy it when you have lost all power yourself. Essentially, it was about the power of words.

Kathleen

The CEO of the Murdoch Children's Research Institute, Dr Terry Dwyer, was listening intently to what I had to say. It was 23 August 2011 and I'd been looking forward to this meeting. I'd planned my words carefully because I knew his response mattered. Not just for me, but for the small group of children worldwide afflicted with the rare neuro-genetic condition known as Angelman Syndrome (AS)

Named after an English paediatrician, Dr Harry Angelman, this little-known syndrome, thought to occur in about one in 20,000 births, is characterised by intellectual disability, sleep disturbance, an unstable, jerky gait and seizures. As if to compensate for their difficult lot in life, these children tend to have happy natures and are known fondly as 'Angels'.

My grandson, Jack, is an Angel. Soon after his birth we knew something wasn't right. He was unable to suck properly and seemed a tiny baby for too long a time, especially compared to his bonny brother and sister. It took a long time to find out what was wrong with him and the diagnosis was devastating when it arrived. He might never walk, would certainly never talk, and would need carers all his life due to mental impairment.

We were told there was no cure. It was almost more than I could bear, but I have a long history of not accepting the inevitable. To me, 'there is no cure' just means we have to find one. And my meeting with Terry Dwyer was part of my plan to do just that. This attitude was to characterise my post-stroke life, and thank goodness for it. I was repeatedly told all the things I wasn't ever going to do, have or be again, but, just as with the prognosis on Angelman Syndrome, I have definitely failed to listen! What you believe tends to become a self-fulfilling prophecy and I knew from the first that the 'no cure' message would be of little benefit.

Cures are brought about by willpower and determination, which takes me to money and research. I believed that some of the methods that I used in the corporate world could be utilised to help find a cure for Angelman Syndrome. Firstly, I knew that Angelman Syndrome has strong links with Alzheimer's disease. At the time, this seemed to be a good thing, as Alzheimer's attracts a lot of funding. What, I wondered, if we could divert some of that money into Angelman's?

It just so happened that Melbourne was due to host an international conference on Alzheimer's in March 2012, about six months after my meeting with Dr Dwyer. I knew that if we could have a session on Angelman Syndrome at that conference, we could start to raise awareness. If he could encourage people to attend, I could use my skills to build discussion and goal setting between people from all around the world to accelerate research and awareness.

I was in my early sixties and in the middle of a busy professional career, built on helping major corporations, and also individuals, plan for the future. I helped them to learn to articulate their problems, think laterally and search widely for solutions. I consulted across Australia and in several other countries. I was busy to the point of being frantic (something I now look back on and wonder if it cost me dearly).

I specialised in events that brought company directors in touch with all levels of the corporation — everyone equally — to work and plan together. This created a dynamic where everyone could focus and work together. If Terry would include Angelman Syndrome at this crucial conference, I could facilitate a session to raise awareness, funding and research. Australia had been sadly absent in the research of this syndrome. Our goal was to send a young Australian postdoctoral researcher to the University of Florida, to work with Dr Edwin J Weeber, whose work with mice was showing great promise.

So the meeting mattered. I was there as the grandmother of an Angel, as someone with useful professional business experience and as a potential future member of the board of the Foundation for Angelman Syndrome Therapeutics (FAST), Australia.

I remember starting to speak, all fired up with ideas and determined to get a result. But how far did we get into that conversation? At what point did the stroke intervene and the talking stop? All I recall is that we discussed enough for me to sense Terry's interest. At some point, I felt dizzy and the room started to spin. I wanted to tell Terry what was happening, to explain why I was faltering. My vision was also deteriorating and I could no longer see him properly all the time — I wasn't even sure he was still in the room.

But I wasn't going to let a temporary dizziness ambush our discussion. Nevertheless, no doubt against my protestations that I was fine, Terry called an ambulance and in doing so probably saved my life. I think I collapsed to the floor. Perhaps I did. Perhaps I didn't. It's not important. Like so many others, this memory no longer exists for me.

But there is one moment that stands out in my mind. It was Terry saying to me, quite calmly, 'Kathleen I'm really interested in this conversation. I would like us to resume it when you're well enough.' He must surely have suspected what was happening to me. He is a doctor and I was having a stroke. But he spoke the words that I so desperately wanted to hear.

Part of me thought, I'll be back! We'll reschedule the meeting and get Angelman Syndrome into the conference. Of course, that didn't happen. But what *did* happen was also significant. His words reminded me that I was a human being and I had made a difference. I clung to them in the months after, and still feel warmed by them. He had observed, understood and spoken to me as a human, not as a medical emergency. In effect, as I read it, he had taken the time to say, *Kathleen, you are still here, you are still Kathleen Jordan, and what mattered to you when you walked into this room, still matters. It has not changed. It has not been negated by illness, nor have you been negated as a human being. Don't give up hope. You will be back.*

As I was to learn, in illness, we are so often reduced to being the sum of our symptoms, tests and scans and not of our individual attributes and personhood.

With Terry's words, I think a part of me felt it could let go. My burden, the message for Angelman Syndrome, had been handed over. But I was disappearing fast. I remember hearing an ambulance officer saying that they needed to get me into the ambulance straight away. And then in the ambulance, for that endless and confused few minutes, priceless kindness. I scarcely knew who I was any longer, and this person — a stranger — was giving me the gift of his whole self, his humanity as well as his care.

I sometimes wonder what the outcome would have been if I had been at home, or perhaps driving towards the meeting, when it all started. Or if I had been alone in the night. These are things all stroke patients wonder about — what went well and what didn't. In time, we can usually find out some answers. But the hardest question has no answer: What could have been?

In that ambulance, I heard the last real words and acts of kindness that I can recall for ages, other than those from my family. Partly that's because I was to drift in and out of consciousness for a long time, but also because I was about to be processed as a stroke victim and that didn't always include kind words. Sometimes it didn't even include being observed, other than for my symptoms and even then in a cursory manner. What they were looking for was disconnected from the person within.

I was about to become a stranger, being treated by strangers. At times I will be a difficult stranger. This is the nature of much illness, particularly brain injury. But when someone takes a moment, as Terry did, to think what this person would want to hear and then articulate it, that's strong medicine indeed. It enters the soul and bolsters the will to live.

The emergency ward of the Royal Melbourne Hospital is noisy, bewilderingly noisy. I can't ever remember hearing noise like this before. It's coming from inside my brain and is all around. Clatter, voices, banging, footsteps, words that boom and echo. It's like I've entered a screaming universe that is overwhelming my brain. This heightened awareness of sound is common in brain injury, but I'm too early into my journey to know that. Inside the cacophony, I lie on my trolley, more alone than I have ever been before. Others lie beside me — I can hear people shouting at them too. We all wait in distress.

I hear someone say that my daughter Lucinda is on her way. Terry Dwyer's colleague had phoned her. My other daughter Emma, who lives away from Melbourne, is being told, as are my four sisters and their families. I sense the shock I have just injected into their day but I long to see them. Knowing they're on their way comforts me like a lifeline through my fog of fear.

But the early stage of stroke is an endless cycle of panic. Nobody knows what is happening or where it will end. The emergency team clusters around. I keep telling myself — and them — that it's just another silly dizzy spell. Do these people know who I am? Am I sure I do? And, foolishly but insistently, the thought keeps badgering me, who will tell my appointments for tomorrow that I may not be there?

I am helpless as a child, unable to save myself as if I was drowning alone in the ocean. The tides of fate are washing over me and unseen forces are in control. I, who have always prided myself on being the person in command, now scarcely know where I am. My head aches and my left arm seems, painfully, to be out of my control. I'm dizzy and nauseous and I still can't see properly. The noise is terrifying; people shouting, machines beeping, things banging and distress all around. Surrounded by strangers, I desperately need someone who knows me.

'Not For Resuscitation'

No amount of education prepares you for the moment when you're told that your loved family member has had a stroke. Or for the moment when medical authorities tell you to prepare for the worst, and it seems like you are absolutely without any power, without volition. Fate is in the driving seat. What should a family do? Accept uncertainty or get involved?

Lucinda

As phones ring, the news of my admission spreads in my family. Shocked, they make their way towards the hospital. Unlike me, they know this isn't just another dizzy spell, but it's too early to know how serious it is. My family contains educated, articulate people. Some of them also have medical training, but faced with this situation they are just like any other family; caught off guard, they're launched into a world they are not prepared for and have little real idea about. They are stunned by the extent to which this proves to be the case.

It now becomes their story, at least for the next few weeks and months. I've pieced it together from what they have told me since, from their memories and emails they sent to each other in that time. When my memories do intrude, they are often nightmarish, with only a slim connection to reality. But to me, that was reality. I've never felt so sure about reality since.

What they have to say makes me uneasy, even after all this

time. They suffered, and I suffer for what they went through, for the anguish that I can't help feeling responsible for. Part of my recovery will be coming to terms with this, and part of their recovery will be assimilating what happened and adjusting.

At the time of my admission, my family consisted of my parents, my two daughters, Emma and Lucinda, and my four sisters. They and their partners were to be my lifeline (not that I was always conscious of the fact) for the next few weeks and then beyond into the years ahead. But as they made their way to the hospital, they could not have known the sort of journey they were in for and what would be asked of them. None of us could have foreseen it.

When my daughter Lucinda reaches the hospital, she desperately tries to get into the emergency ward to see me, but is stopped by the triage nurse who tells her to wait in line. Through the window behind her, Lucinda can see me and explains to the nurse that she is terrified that her mother is about to die. She is told to wait yet again. The nurse turns back to the elderly man who is arguing about his bill, a controversy that seems to be going in circles. After some time, other people also queuing for triage see her distress at not being allowed to get through. So she can get to me, they stand aside to offer her their place in the queue.

In the ward, there is little time for family members to face their own shock and grief. My condition has started to deteriorate. When I was first admitted, the nurse had asked me my weight and I'd quipped 'too much'. But I'm now beyond humour and my speech is slurred. I'm frightened and not always sure that my family really is here with me or if I just think they are. I drift in and out of consciousness.

In truth, I'm in more need of help than a busy ward can offer. My family is left on its own in the vast, crowded emergency department, trying to bolster each other, and keep me calm, all the while wondering what's in store. As someone recalls, 'Things seemed to be becoming very dire indeed. There were hours of confusion for the family, and decreasing consciousness for Kathleen. It was all very negative and confused.'

They are kept busy, gratefully drawing on the nursing skills of my sister to ensure I'm receiving basic care. When I vomit, they clear my mouth and wipe my face, placing me on my side so I don't choke. My mouth is terribly dry and they moisten it with a large swab, but my thirst is unquenchable. I reach out and grab the swab from them, then start sawing it in and out so clumsily they have to take it away from me. When I'm able to, I ask questions they don't know the answers to. In the face of my increasing fear ('What's happening? I don't know what's happening!') they have nothing to calm me with other than their presence.

What I don't know is that the results are coming in from my scan. My 'dizzy spell' is a major right haemorrhagic stroke, a particularly dangerous medical scenario which few survive. The CT scan describes it as 'a large right sided intracranial haemorrhage extending from the basal ganglia through the centrum semiovale. Within this there is a central spherical 2x2cm hypodensity, possibly hyperacute non-clotted blood or a mass legion. There is intraventricular extension. There is mass effect of 7mm of midline shift and effacement of the anterior horn of the right lateral ventricle. The temporal horn of the left lateral ventricle is prominent and may represent early hydrocephalus. Periventricular white matter low attenuation is consistent with chronic small vessel ischaemic change.'

Stroke occurs four times more frequently in the left cerebral hemisphere than the right, and 83 per cent of strokes are ischaemic, that is, caused by a blood clot blocking the blood and oxygen flow to the cells. So the fact that I have a right side haemorrhagic stroke, with blood flooding into the brain from a ruptured blood vessel, means that my stroke is significantly more serious and less predictable than most.

By the time my sister Petrina, a general practitioner, arrives, the other family members have been taken into a room with the neurology registrar. This is the long awaited moment, when answers are expected. What they hear shocks them. Petrina explains:

I arrived to a number of people sitting in a meeting with the neurology registrar. He was midway into explaining to the family members, that Kathleen had had a stroke, that it was haemorrhagic and they weren't going to operate. He showed us the scan so we could see where the haemorrhage was. I knew, as a doctor, that this was not good news. If it had been a blockage, they would have been able to give her medication to dissolve the clot.

To our shock, the registrar then started to have a NFR (Not For Resuscitation) discussion with us. I was very surprised. It was not really a discussion but presented to us as a fait accompli. He told us that given the size of the haemorrhage, should she survive, Kathleen would be unlikely to have any quality of life. She would either be very dependent and live in a nursing home or else live the rest of her life in a highly vegetative state.

We were not being consulted at all. It sounded like a decision had been made somewhere and it was being presented to us — like he was paying lip service to us in the consultation. I felt totally disempowered by the way he put it.

Petrina realises that this is a critical moment in my care — as indeed it turns out to be. Unable to speak for myself, she feels the need to speak on my behalf, saying, 'I don't suppose this will make any difference, but Kathleen is a very strong person, connected, warm, loving, intelligent, resourceful. She's still young and I don't think she's finished living yet.' And he did seem to take a step back at that point, but he certainly didn't say we'll take off the NFR.

NFR, in this circumstance, means that if there are any further adverse medical events, perhaps a heart attack or another stroke, they will not resuscitate me. I will be looked after, but my life will not be actively saved.

Petrina's words halt the registrar's flow. For the first time, the family's voice is heard — who I am, who we are, what we think. I've been brought into the room as a *person* and not just a medical event.

A collective sigh of relief flows through the room. Petrina has voiced what they were all thinking. The registrar naturally knows nothing about me, other than medically. It may have been just a hope they're clinging to, but my family know me well enough to know I'll never give up. *Ever.* But I need to be given a chance. And that means I need to have full attention focused on my recovery and not to be sidelined by a prognosis that precludes the concept of meaningful recovery.

'At that moment, I was definitely speaking as a sister and not a doctor,' Petrina recalls. 'I felt non-medical when I said that about Kathleen. It was bringing in an emotional aspect, but I was also trying to draw on any medical authority I could muster. I don't think I'd seen her yet, just scans and doctors' opinions. I was thinking it was a terrible scenario but I also thought it was very early days and you could not put a prognosis on her at this stage.'

From that moment, my family sensed an invisible gear change. 'It was like everything ramped up. The system invested in her at last,' recalls a family member. The situation remained confused, but during the night, as my condition deteriorated, I was reassessed for surgery.

Advocacy is a major theme of this book and one of the reasons I wanted to write it. This was my family's first act of advocacy, standing up for a sister who could not do it herself. I think over and over that their request was a simple one, but had they not asked, I'm not sure I'd be here today. They were really asking: Can we stop and talk and think about Kathleen? Can we please not rush to conclusions too early? Please talk to us.

Confusion

We were all in shock. That morning we had an incredibly vibrant and independent woman, and suddenly we are being told that she is unlikely to live and that if she does, she may be bedridden, a vegetable.

Lucinda

As the hours pass, my family starts to assimilate the new reality brought by this hideous day. But beyond the fact that I'm seriously unwell, what is this reality? Will I be operated on or not? *Should* I be operated on? What are the doctors thinking? Answers are hard to come by, but they keep trying from inside their daze, helping each other as best they can.

I'm still in the emergency ward, and they don't know why. The noise never stops, day becomes night and they struggle with despair and fear, unwilling witnesses to the human grief and drama all around. The staff shuttles past from one cubicle to another, busy and preoccupied. There is no place for family here. It was not designed for the people who naturally want to stay close to the bedside of a loved one.

The situation doesn't seem right for someone diagnosed with a stroke. My family's fear is that leaving me here might be part of the medical decision not to resuscitate. After all, why would you bother putting a patient you weren't intending to resuscitate into intensive care? My daughter Lucinda recalls an overwhelming sense that I just wasn't being looked after.

Some family members leave to get sleep, so they can return in the morning. There is little more that can be done or said, other than to stay in touch and make sure I'm not left alone. My elderly parents have yet to be told and one of my sisters departs to share the terrible news with them. The real world is making its brutal way back into everyone's lives.

On hearing the news, my mother, who described me as her beautiful and fun loving eldest daughter, was overcome with grief. 'Not the same grief that overwhelmed me when this vital, lovely daughter left home at 22 years of age. That grief was sprinkled with the joy of sharing, from afar, the new excitement she was finding daily. This grief was *overwhelming*.'

In the emergency ward, my two daughters, Emma and Lucinda, settle in to stay by my side for the night.

Lucinda recalls, 'It was a horrendous evening. There were not many doctors around by then. There were some nurses, but we had this overwhelming sense of Mum not being looked after. She was vomiting and choking and we had to keep running out of her cubicle and shouting for help. *What if we hadn't been there?* Once, we were asked to wait outside the cubicle while a nurse was in with mum and another nurse came along and started shouting at us. What were we doing? We explained why we were there, and then he apologised, explaining that they get people who snoop around. I know there's a lot of stress in those departments, but it was cruel on us.'

Emma says, 'We felt so helpless. We felt something urgently needed to be done. Instead we were waiting … waiting. The inactivity was a distressing contrast to our sense of urgency and emergency. We told Mum everything was OK, reassured her that she was in good hands, *while knowing full well that wasn't the case.* Mum was in a great deal of pain, asleep, awake, then confused. At one point we realised we didn't know if Mum's contact lenses were still in, or had been removed and I found myself adding to her distress as I poked around in her eye, endlessly apologising.'

Adding to Emma and Lucinda's burden of shock is their confusion about what was going to happen to me. They'd heard several conflicting assessments about what the best course of action might be. The registrar's grim pronouncement that I was one of the worst he'd seen and that should I survive the night, it would be to spend my days in a nursing home, is still ringing in their ears.

That registrar had also told them he believed a tumour might have caused my stroke. They'd informed him I'd had a pre-melanoma removed a few weeks previously. Now they fear he has jumped to this conclusion, going straight to, 'Oh she's got brain cancer.' They are far from convinced. They had already been told by another registrar, this one from the neurosurgery department, that it definitely *wasn't* caused by a tumour and, in her view, I shouldn't be operated on because of the size of the bleed and the danger it would pose to my life.

Everyone understands that the situation is evolving and the doctors don't have clarity themselves. A decision that seems right one hour can tip the other way the next. But the lack of clear discussion and direction adds to my daughters' load. They are trying to do the right thing, but feel confused and isolated, with so much at stake. My daughters are clever and caring girls: Emma the devoted and loving older sister, a wonderful mother to her three children. Lucinda filled with strong ideas, committed to social justice and passionately in pursuit of excellence. Known for her thoughtfulness when interviewing people less fortunate than herself for her work and academic writing, Lucinda would never have left people hanging in despair and uncertainty.

But despair and uncertainty for families is not uncommon. In her memoir of brain injury acquired as a result of a car accident, *Doing up Buttons,* Christine Durham explains a similar situation. Her husband had grappled with the medical information given to him about her after the accident and lamented that it remained unclear and incomprehensible throughout her entire hospital stay.

Amidst the uncertainty and lack of medical consensus, my family is most distressed by not knowing if I'm being monitored or assessed sufficiently. Is anyone discussing me at a senior level? If so, are they assessing me without presumptions as to the likely outcome? They may well be. But my family just doesn't know. Nothing is being communicated. The lack of reassurance leaves them understandably frantic. One of my sisters, a neuropsychologist, puts it beautifully, 'We needed to know that they had her best interests at heart. You wouldn't hand over your child unless it's to someone who absolutely cares, and Kathleen was like a child, totally vulnerable.'

Surgery

Head injuries do not happen to individuals,
they happen to whole families.
Tony Moore, author of *Cry of the Damaged Man*

As other family members arrive in the early morning, my daughters leave to get some rest. By now I'm very fearful, speaking in a drawl, neurologically agitated, and my movements are jerky. My left side is paralysed, but I'm still unaware of that. When, some weeks later, I'm told about it, I will deny it vigorously.

No sooner do my exhausted girls reach home than the phone rings. It is the neurosurgeon who tells them I need to be taken into surgery straight away. This is a new turn of events, and a critical one. Lucinda is told there is no choice: without surgery to reduce the swelling, I will die. They need to relieve the pressure in my brain and suck out the blood clot. Otherwise pressure will build up until my brain 'cones', which means it is pushed into the spinal canal as a result of insufficient room inside the skull.

Why now, they wonder? If surgery has suddenly become the best course — in fact the only course — could it also have been the best course earlier? Why was I not taken into surgery soon after arrival? Did the presumption of NFR compromise other decisions?

It's something I still struggle with from time to time: if I had been operated on earlier, would I have more function today and saved myself so many struggles in the following years? We still don't know. Now, of course, it is irrelevant, just part of what happened and I'm grateful for the surgery and the life it undoubtedly gave me.

But for my daughters, being asked to sign the consent for my surgery, these are heavy weights. They are in a poor state to make decisions and of course, no one is ready and in the right state of mind after an emergency. Only hours before, they'd been told quite clearly that surgery would kill me. The implications of what they're being asked to do seem overwhelming. My sister Petrina was finding that even as a medico, it felt very confusing. She wondered if having stuck up for me at the meeting the day before had produced the situation where they said, 'Perhaps we'd better operate.'

My daughters return to the hospital to sign the forms and discuss with the doctors what will be done if I have an adverse event during surgery. Now that the decision to operate has been made, it feels fraught with risk and deeply onerous. But they also feel that finally something is being done.

There is no opportunity for goodbyes. Sedated in readiness for the procedure, I am beyond knowing anything. My daughters kiss me, tell me how much they love me and urge me to hang on. But I look dreadful and they can hardly bear to look at me. Each says goodbye, thinking, 'This could be it.'

Earlier that morning some members of my family had dropped in and been present when the surgeons made the decision that they needed to operate. My brother-in-law, Gordon, on his way to work, found me unconscious but not yet sedated for intubation in readiness for surgery. Realising that this meant he would need to deputise for the family, he kissed me goodbye, hoping that I would feel his love and hear his words of strength.

As the surgery progresses, many family members gather at the hospital, preparing for the worst. My parents, frail in their walking frames, wait with their four daughters as their eldest undergoes surgery. Seventeen years older than my youngest sibling, Petrina, I was always known as the daughter who could cope and manage everything. 'If there's a problem, Kathleen will solve it,' my mother always said. Now I am the vulnerable one, to an extent they could never have imagined.

It is late afternoon when they hear that I'm in recovery. Riding the lift up to ICU, my daughter Emma clearly remembers the depth of her fear. She had spent the day consciously holding a candle of hope for me in her mind. Lucinda recalls being so shocked and tired by the whole event, so certain that I was going to die, that when told I was in recovery she only felt confusion. 'I had to ask, does that mean Mum's survived? Is it *good* that she's in recovery?'

Two at a time, they come and stand by my bed. In an induced coma, wired up to monitors, intravenous drips and breathing apparatus, my head partially shaved, I look both peaceful and hellishly confronting. My mother holds me as much as is possible, and whispers, 'Hold on Kathleen. You are very, very precious.' The surgeon, who everyone remembers for his kindness, spends time explaining. My life has been saved, the surgery has gone as well as could be hoped for, but the right side of my brain was damaged by the stroke and surgery. As a result, my whole left side is paralysed. I may or may not recover. I may be in a vegetative state for life.

Exhaustion and relief that I am, at least, alive, fills my family. Tomorrow can't be thought about right now. What matters is that I have been given a chance and am no longer captive to a grim prognosis that didn't include a worthwhile future. Huge effort and skill have been expended to help me live. To everyone's enormous relief, I have left the chaos of the emergency ward far behind.

Knowing that in intensive care I will be watched over by a specialist nurse 24 hours a day finally allows everyone to return home in the knowledge that I am being cared for to the fullest possible extent.

As they leave, each looks back with a private thought. Seeing the nurse, the monitors tracing my every signal and the staff surrounding me, Emma feels a wave of reassurance.

Petrina, knowing that my future is far from certain, walks over to talk to the ICU nurses. As in the first meeting with the registrar, she senses that if she can tell them about me, turn me into a person and not just a disabled body, it may help: 'Probably I still feared there was a danger of the medical team writing Kathleen off, as had seemed to happen in the emergency department.' So Petrina tells them about me, my work, my advocacy on Angelman Syndrome and she senses that they are interested. She also senses that despite my situation I am very much 'still in there' as her sister. The next challenge will be to return myself to myself.

Everything that can be done has now been done and the turmoil of the past 36 hours is slowing into steady acceptance. Relieved of the immediate burden, a new journey begins for my family, mostly around waiting and hoping. In their hearts, they wonder what is going to happen next and what my real capacity for recovery will be.

Afterwards

Despite the predictions and everyone's worst fears, I delighted everyone with an early recovery in intensive care. Not only was I still there, I was still the same mum, sister and daughter they had known. Seeing me in a light room, away from the chaos of the emergency department, they felt that I was now 'in good hands.' But the aftermath of stroke isn't necessarily a straight progression. Hopes that are raised are soon dashed.

Kathleen

The next morning, my family wakes to the news that I am also awake. 'She was awake!' says Lucinda. 'It was so great when we got the call and so exciting when she opened her eyes. Then there was quite an improvement after the first 24 hours. We were really excited as we began to realise that she was *still there.*

'At first she had tubes down her throat and couldn't talk. She began to wave her right arm around and we realised, eventually, that she wanted to write. So we found a pen and paper and then she was writing things like her appointments, the name of different people, the need to cancel some meetings. She was back to bossy Kathleen! And we were able to say, "Don't worry, we've read your diary and it's all being taken care of."'

The realisation that my arm waving isn't just more physical agitation, but a poorly relayed message, leads to great hope.

While they know these early situations need to be measured in hours and minutes, they can't help but be excited by the positive news. 'Once she'd survived, that was everything and you just go on with hope from that point,' says Lucinda. 'To be honest, we presumed she was going to die, so surviving surgery was massive. Then, each little thing became exciting — opening her eyes, trying to write, telling my uncle she couldn't move one side.'

They can't believe that one of my first acts is to try to communicate. It makes them aware of the need to watch me carefully, to understand what might be going on. Over the next months, this awareness will be a critical part of my recovery. They will watch and notice what the medical staff, rushed off their feet, simply don't have time to do.

The relief for me of being able to convey my thoughts is wonderful. I had been so frustrated at not being able to communicate. 'We thought it was hilarious that she was writing *instructions* to us,' Emma recalls. 'She had looked so fragile, connected to all those things, and we'd had such trepidation about the surgery, and so many fears for her. Afterwards there was joy when she became conscious.'

My oldest friend, Liz, arrives back from Singapore, having been told of my stroke. Unaware of the severity, she heads straight to the hospital from the airport. 'I got the shock of my life. It was about two days after Kathleen's stroke. She was in intensive care with half her head shaved, tubes everywhere, linked up to machines. It was an incredible shock to see a woman who always had thick lustrous hair, lying there with electrodes everywhere. But, as serious as it was, when she saw me walking towards her and recognised me, her eyes lit up. She knew I was there.'

Miraculously, I also begin to speak a few words. Watching this prompts my family to put even more effort into helping me recover quickly. They stay by my side, talk to me, to the nurses and to each other. They are wonderful. Nobody could ask for more.

They also read what they can about my condition, but find useful information elusive. Often they feel they are working on their own, without the assistance they need at this critical time. Petrina decides she must spend as much time as possible with me. That way, she will hear the decisions as they're being made and see the doctors' faces. Her aim is to monitor the medical side of my situation. She asks the nurses many questions and, by her own admission, really grills the doctors. She knows that you might miss out if you're not there at the times of the doctors' rounds.

Petrina becomes the conduit between that medical information and the family, who wait for her explanations. One very good intern tries everything he can to relay what the medical team think and answer questions. But he is one person. The lack of ongoing information is a constant anxiety. What is discussed this week no longer feels adequate the next. They want to know that everyone is on the same page, that they've been heard, that I'm being constantly reviewed and considered in light of my changes.

And the changes appear quickly. My early burst of communication ebbs, to be replaced with silence and weak response. I am moved into a high dependency unit, one step down from intensive care, but still with full time observation and care. But to everyone's dismay, my level of consciousness remains low. My brother-in-law Mark notices nurses having to pinch me and thump heavily on my chest to arouse me. What has happened?

Petrina notices a link between my level of responsiveness and the temporary shunt, which was inserted during surgery, being clamped off. 'Kathleen would be responding to commands such as "move your hands", maybe even talking a little and then they'd clamp off the tube and she'd go flat as pressure built up in her brain,' she recalls. 'I noticed this a couple of times — it seemed very marked to me.'

She speaks to the nursing staff to find out *why* it is being closed off but emerges from the conversations 'never totally sure of their explanation.' She decides to ring the neurosurgeon directly, and soon after a second craniotomy is performed, in which a permanent shunt is installed.

'It wouldn't be normal to call him,' says Petrina. 'The only reason I could speak to him was that I was a GP, I think. Kathleen was also feverish and, after having the infectious diseases people look at her, they decided it was ventriculitis, which is inflammation or infection of the ventricles of the brain.' After treatment with antibiotics, I start to improve.

The bed next to mine is occupied by a noisy and emotionally disinhibited man, who is testing everyone's patience. When nurses come to ask me questions designed to assess my level of awareness, he cheerfully takes it upon himself to answer on my behalf. When they ask if I know where I am, he answers loudly through the curtains, 'Royal Melbourne Hospital.'

All I have to do is repeat his answers, which is easy for me, but makes it hard for anyone to get a private word or sense of my true state. He also starts bombarding nurses with obscene suggestions and captures my family visitors with questions on their lives and past. One day, after some of his more trying interjections I have a rare moment of lucidity. I turn to my visitor, who happens to be my future son-in-law, Richard, and tell him, quite clearly, that he has my permission to punch my neighbour's lights out!

But it's a rare moment. My conscious state remains impaired — a possible side effect of the surgery they are told, or maybe my extreme tiredness is simply a part of the normal process of haemorrhagic stroke. They just don't know.

By the time I move into the stroke unit, I am rarely speaking. My brother-in-law Mark recalls the situation. 'We were working on the today, the here and now, working out who was going to be sitting with Kathleen. This consumed our time. And we were all doing our own homework, trying to put the pieces of the jigsaw together, talking to colleagues. Really trying to understand what the hell was going on.'

The stroke unit

I remember on the stroke unit, feeling so relieved my family was keeping vigil. My brother-in-law Mark was there almost every day, as were my sisters. I couldn't communicate with them much, but there was great comfort from their presence, lots of hugs, kisses and touch.

Kathleen

When the person you love is unconscious, and you're not sure if it's part of their recovery or part of their deterioration, what do you do? This is the situation that faced my family: the first phase of the waiting game where the future unfolds slowly and uncertainly.

They decide the best way is to ensure that everything humanly possible is done to aid my recovery. Whatever is happening inside my brain is opaque to everyone, but who knows what will tip the balance? Perhaps just being there, watching, able to intervene when needed, any small action, may be the one revealed as having been important.

Their mission is to be with me, to make sure that someone is by my side during as many daylight hours as possible. Of course they want to be there, but there's a practical purpose too, watching over my care, speaking to medical staff, observing my progress and encouraging my recovery in every way possible. They create a system of continuous practical and emotional support.

It takes a bit of organisation. At first, family members arrive and sometimes need to stay in the waiting room while others are with me. An orderly process is needed to ensure it all works efficiently and it is my future son-in-law, Richard, who comes up with the idea of an internet-based roster. This roster becomes the communications lifeline of the family, allowing people to slot in the times they're available and see at a glance when others are here with me.

It is also the basis for rapid feedback. Did Kathleen speak this afternoon? What did she say? Was there any improvement? What are the doctors saying? Any grains of information are eagerly sought and shared, allowing those like my daughter Emma, in Warrnambool with a young family, to be part of the care even from home. Every weekend she drives to Melbourne. 'When such big things are happening in the family, we all really just wanted to be together. For me that wasn't possible, other than on weekends. So what really helped, apart from being physically present, were the constant emails and texts that kept us all up-to-date.'

Lucinda recalls being surprised by how much time everyone wanted to put in. 'To be with her was incredibly important for everyone. We wanted to have someone with her, keeping watch. To enable that, we sent constant emails back and forth, reporting every day on what had happened, what the latest was.'

They persist, but generally receive little response from me for their efforts. Their presence was a huge comfort, even though I couldn't say at what level I was conscious of it. I may have appeared unresponsive, yet my dominant memory is of their care and comfort. It was a critical part of coming back to myself again.

Mark, who just happened not to be working during these hospital weeks and who lived nearby, spent many hours with me as part of the family schedule. Knowing how gregarious I am and how much I love people, gardens and the sunlight, he decided, one day, to take me out of the hospital to experience those things again. Getting out will do me good!

'I felt Kathleen needed to get out, get some sunshine,' he recounts. 'She had metal stitches in her head but I thought I'll take her out along Sydney Road. I put her in her wheelchair, wrapped a sheet over her and off we set, out along Royal Parade, left into Story Street, Park Drive and back along Flemington Road and Grattan Street. We were both a bit daunted. I took a white hospital blanket with me and I can recall thinking how easy it was to do a runner with an RMH patient — no-one challenged me when we left the ward or the hospital entrance. I could have taken her anywhere!

'It was quite a struggle holding on in the downhill stretch along Park Drive — it was hard work and at one stage I thought I was going to lose her! But I had her laughing. She always had a great sense of humour and she responded to that and she enjoyed the warmth of the sun on her body so much that we did this on most visits.' Even now, the image of both us as escapees, with Mark struggling behind my runaway wheelchair, makes me laugh.

But these adventures were an exciting interlude in the midst of not very much. 'There were many times we sat around holding her hand and feeling a bit useless,' one of my sisters recalls. Most visits are simply about keeping vigil while I sleep. They try speaking to me, sometimes massaging my left side, rubbing my skin with moisturisers and repositioning me as I constantly slump to the right, as a result of paralysis down my left side. They also try straightening my left arm, fingers and leg to prevent them getting contractures. Sometimes they read to me. Later, when my naso-gastric tube is removed, they help me eat.

They watch the nursing. Knowing the nurses are pressed for time (that's the system), they try to make sure I'm not too adversely affected. They have plenty of opportunities. One day, after a gap in the roster, Petrina and Gordon arrive to find me sitting in a chair and realise I've been in it for six hours. I'd been forgotten. Only when told do the nurses realise their mistake. I'm being encouraged to sit up by the physios, but this marathon has left me exhausted. It reinforces everyone's belief that without a strong family presence and advocacy, I'm unlikely to recover as well as I could.

'It's being there to watch these things, to swab her mouth, or to call the nurses and say it really is time to change that incontinence pad,' one of my sisters, a nurse herself, explains. She speaks to the unit manager about my level of nursing, feeling some of it is substandard, but aware of how short-staffed these places are. Her desire for me to be kept dry, hydrated and comfortable seems fairly basic, but often proves elusive.

In fact, just ensuring that I'm kept dry while incontinent is a major concern. I've always been a person of great dignity, fastidious in dress and grooming. In the face of many unthinking violations of my dignity they ask, 'Why should personal dignity matter less after a stroke?' When I'm slowly regaining continence, I ask the nurse to bring me a bedpan, but she's busy so shouts over to me, 'Just do it in the bed.' It was one occasion, but we were all shocked.

My family ensures that curtains are pulled around when I'm being undressed and that my incontinence is attended to quickly. 'It was a huge thing — making sure Kathleen was changed regularly,' Emma recalls. 'Some weekends I'd drive all the way down to see her and she'd be in and out of consciousness and none the wiser that I'd been there. But it was important to me to ensure that the care, especially around dignity, was there when she needed it. It felt really important to be there, and keep reminding them of her need for dignity.'

Dignity involves many things. My inability to govern my own behaviour raises issues regarding visits from friends and colleagues, as I yawn widely without covering my mouth and I don't notice when my clothing slips. I am what is known as disinhibited following the trauma to my brain. Given a choice, I wouldn't want anyone to see me like this.

They make a difficult decision, based on my best interests, and firmly request no visits from friends and colleagues. Instead, they keep them informed by text, phone and email. They explain, 'We felt part of our vigilance was to protect Kathleen from visitors, other than close family and her closest friends.' For several weeks they field calls and queries (constantly, according to Lucinda), but they know I'm not ready yet to see people. It's a decision that's validated when one person turns up to see me just as I'm pulling my clothes off.

Friends and colleagues quickly adjust, respecting the family decision and not wanting to add to Lucinda and Emma's burdens. They appreciate the information and calls they receive and await the day I'll be well enough to see them. In time, they too will play a critical role in my recovery.

More silence

Despite my family's efforts, I remain difficult to rouse in the weeks after surgery. My frequent sighing, big deep sighs, alerts my family to the possibility that I might be depressed and I start being given anti-depressant medication which is known to improve the outcome in stroke. Hoists are needed to move me about and I'm fed through a naso-gastric tube.

I am clearly the most incapacitated of all the patients in the stroke unit. My family, as they walk past the now familiar surrounds of ICU, still feel some measure of comfort that I have at least progressed beyond that balance between life and death. But why have I stopped talking? Why am I non-responsive?

When I do wake, I'm frequently very distressed, but unable to tell anyone why. Everyone's relief following surgery, when I was blithely issuing instructions (albeit written), and then my spoken (albeit confused) words in the high dependency unit, gives way to real concern over my continuing muteness. Answers are hard to find. My neuropsychologist sister recalls, 'No-one ever came out and said, the reason Kathleen isn't talking is ... A speech therapist thought she might have oral apraxia (an inability to speak due to damage to the brain) but they didn't seem to really know.'

The speech therapist, acting on this assumption, tries to teach me to copy sounds. But the decision to treat my silence as apraxia seems misguided to my sister. Increasingly, and in consultation with her peers, she believes my problem is due to disruption of deep centres in the brain and their cortical connections, and that lack of speech was due to my general problems of arousal. 'Really, we can now see the reason Kathleen wasn't talking was because she'd had a massive stroke and her brain was so addled. Even though she *should* have been talking (because she had a right side stroke and language is in the left hemisphere), there just wasn't enough cerebral activation going on for her to be having these higher-level cognitive processes. She was in survival mode. Her brain and body were just focusing on bodily functions.'

She believes I would benefit from neuropsychological involvement. Looking back at that time, she says, 'Neuropsychological involvement in the stroke unit would have been so helpful to guide the therapy, support the family and advocate for Kathleen. Kathleen was getting nursing care, including physiotherapy (around support and endurance for sitting), occupational therapy (for one-handed strategies for grooming and starting to scan to the left) and speech therapy (for lip sealing and swallowing). But a neuropsychologist would have helped make sure that what was being done was most beneficial.

'For example, given Kathleen's lack of speech and her left-side neglect, we developed our own communication device — a list of single words, such as *yes, no, headache* which we wrote in a column on the right side of the page for Kathleen to point to. We needed a way of understanding the reasons behind her frequent and obvious distress so that we could help. She was able to use this simple device with some success.'

'We can say this with some clarity now, but when you're in the thick of it, you've got questions and there are no answers. Sometimes that's because there are no answers, or there is no access to people who may have the answers. Really, the staff are trying to put the pieces together themselves and even those who were really well intentioned saw it as their duty, I think, to keep us grounded. Things were bad and were going to stay bad for a very long time, if not forever. Their main focus, as they saw it, was to not raise our expectations. But that didn't help us at all.'

Other people's modest expectations have to be brushed aside if my family are to believe I will get through this. And that is what they do. Guided by their own inner convictions and knowledge of what a determined survivor I've been all my life, they get on with providing me the company and stimulation they think I need. They chat away to me, even though I don't reply. They talk, letting me know they're there. In my memory (and it's backed up by email correspondence), they are always there.

Mark found the best way to communicate during my silence was to sit by my bedside and simply embark on a monologue of his own. It was his brand of cheerful companionship, letting me know that I was still in their lives, but he chatted without expectation of response. Mostly I relaxed at the sound of his voice, but one of his monologues must have gone on too long, even for a bedridden mute. When it concluded, I looked at him and told him that he was driving me up the wall. He took it as a good sign!

In late September, a month after the stroke, Lucinda was able to email everyone that I had spoken a complete sentence. Unfortunately, it wasn't the best one! Reflective of my limited insight into where I was and what had happened, I turned to my lovely, deeply distressed daughter and said, 'What a wonderful year you are having, darling!' She bit back the obvious, ironic reply.

The police arrive

When eventually, I do begin to speak, it's quickly apparent that something isn't right. I ask my family to pass me that cup of tea, or to fetch some of the ginger beer that I keep in the fridge. None of it exists. Feverish, I throw my covers off, alarming my family afresh with my thoughts and behaviour. I had made some progress, conquering the ability to swallow, which allowed my naso-gastric tube to be removed. But the strange things I tell them start to overshadow the progress.

I am convinced, absolutely, that the Royal Melbourne Hospital is being built over my house. Not my current house, which I'm unable to recall, but a tiny one in Kew that I had owned many years ago. In outrage, I tell Mark about the scaffolding they've erected around my bed and demand that he goes to hospital management right now and get it taken down. It's a difficult situation. As Mark says, 'Woe betides anyone who contradicted her. Such treachery. And this delusion was just the beginning!'

I call the consultants vandals for what they've done to my home. I tell one of my sisters that it must be awful to bring Mum and Dad to see me in my home with this hospital built around it. There is no rhyme or reason to what I say, but it gets worse.

I start to believe that I have, unwittingly, become part of a paedophile ring and am being chased by the police. This is due to an online dating service and the Royal Melbourne Hospital colluding to run a paedophile ring. Somehow, I've become caught up in this dreadful situation. The sound of an ambulance siren (there are many near a major hospital) sends me into a state of terror as I try to escape the police who I believe are coming for me.

Trying to make sense of it now, I believe I must have seen a television programme on the prevalence of paedophilia just before my stroke and it was almost like a dream on replay. Or perhaps it was because I had seen my little grandchildren brought in by Emma, and my love for them and the unknown fears I was feeling for myself, intersected in the unfathomable way of the brain. Whatever the cause, it took years for the sound of a siren not to send me into terror. I needed to steel myself and say firmly, 'Kathleen, it's just a police car and you haven't done anything wrong.'

It becomes another issue of dignity. Knowing how I'd hate to be seen in this state, my family remove my phone to ensure I don't make any bizarre phone calls. They continue to keep friends at a distance.

I feel, in my rare lucid moments, that I've lost myself completely. I struggle with noise. I struggle with nurses who don't make an effort to understand me. I struggle to remember who I was and who I am. Days whirl around and even at my clearest I'm bewildered. If I'm living through a nightmare of illusions, then perhaps it's because this is not a nightmare at all, but my waking reality.

I remain psychotic for months. As I move out of the hospital nine weeks after the stroke and into the rehabilitation unit, I'm still raving. My argumentative stance and stubborn beliefs make it even harder for my family. I must have been hard to love.

'If you disagreed with her, you'd get your head bitten off,'

Petrina says. The best approach, they find, is to sympathise with my version of events without actually colluding. But I want more than sympathy and feel increasingly distressed that they're not doing what I want them to. Their attempts to placate me don't work. One of my sisters, trying to awaken my trust, says, 'Kathleen, I'm your sister. Don't you trust me?' I reply firstly, with a 'yes'. She asks me again and this time I reply with 'possibly', and the third time, only 'perhaps'. It's a shattering realisation that these weeks of support and constant presence are not bringing me peace.

My psychotic phase has interludes and, as usual, humour is the true measure of my mental state. One day I turn to Lucinda and say, 'Oh, look at that statue floating in the air. Isn't it beautiful?' Lucinda replies, 'Mum, there is no statue' and suddenly we're laughing. I agree that a floating statue does sound rather peculiar. On another occasion I observe Richard slumped with exhaustion on the end of my bed. 'He has been shooting up again?' I ask Lucinda suspiciously. 'Yeah, of course mum,' she replies deadpan, 'that's exactly what he's been up to.' The happy ending to that observation is that we both collapsed laughing again. Even I must have realised how ridiculous it was.

For Lucinda, those moments of humour were reassuring. 'They were really important during that time, and gave us a positive way of interacting with her. They also helped to take her away from the scary thoughts she was having.'

My psychosis first became apparent in the stroke unit. Again, it was family, rather than staff, who noticed it. As the paranoid I had become, I was careful in whom I confided my fears. So my family heard what others didn't. Thank goodness they were there. At home they each read and shared articles, trying to find an answer to my puzzling descent into psychosis.

The depression that I'm being treated for is common after stroke but psychosis is more rare. It's a double worry for my family. Obviously, they worry about my behaviour and what has gone wrong to create it. But they also worry that my impaired mental state is retarding my recovery. These early weeks are critical weeks in the rehabilitation process. I'm about to move into the rehabilitation unit, but how can I be expected to start rehabilitation unless I can understand what is being said to me? How can I be expected to respond appropriately? Will I be seen as unresponsive because I don't really know what's going on?

It's a bit easier for me. In my deluded state, I've convinced myself that my disability is less real than it is — a classic instance of mistaking my delusions for reality. In fact, I don't really believe I have much of a problem and so naturally that makes me a bit blasé about making an effort. Rehab, huh! That's for the birds.

My family, ever watchful, hunts for answers. They are unsure exactly where I am in the recovery process. Is this sort of psychotic behaviour part of post-stroke recovery? Is it telling them something about my brain that they don't yet understand the importance of? Has the shunt surgery damaged my brain?

When they decide to step in and get an assessment on my mental state, they discover there is no access to a psychiatric consultant in rehab. Undeterred, they contact a family friend who is a psychiatrist and she sends a colleague to visit me. I am given medication to treat the psychosis.

It confirms what my family now know only too well. You watch your loved one and make your own decisions. Just because a trained member of staff hasn't noticed something, doesn't mean it doesn't exist. Staff look for a set of predetermined events or outcomes because that's what they're trained to do and what occurs outside their field of vision may not be noticed. We all see what we're looking for. So, a family must watch and take action where appropriate to get what is needed for their loved one. How much longer would this damaging psychosis have prevented me from participating in rehab if they hadn't intervened? Could my psychosis have been mistaken for a permanent psychological change?

They tread wearily forward. Nobody can tell them much and after this unexpected episode, they scarcely now know the questions to ask. They long for someone to say, 'Don't worry too much, this is a normal phase, all things considered' but the medical opinion, when they seek it, keeps their expectations low. Perhaps it's a form of kindness, and perhaps it's good advice. But if you aim low, what possibilities can be missed?

Slow battles of fast-stream rehab

The sub-acute rehabilitation ward is where my interaction with life starts again. It's a shaky start. Still psychotic, but starting to talk, I confidently explain my room's location to everyone who visits. 'It's on the top floor above the main area of the unit — just go up the stairs,' I tell them, and they arrive to find there is no top floor. It's a rehab unit! Of course there are no stairs!

More sinisterly, I also believe that people are swapping my room about. Whoever is behind this ruse is going to a lot of effort, as my walls are covered with cards from friends and messages of inspiration. The person who is moving me is also moving these cards and taking enormous care to place them exactly as they were. But they can't trick me, I'm on to them!

Having your room invaded by unknown people who don't have your best interests at heart is frightening and confusing. And nobody believes me. My first weeks in rehab are dark and sinister.

'Kathleen expressed frustration and sadness about being moved into different rooms,' my psychologist writes in my therapy book on October 27 2011. This little exercise book, which rapidly becomes fragile with use, lies beside my bed and is written in by everyone — family, nurses and therapists, even me — during my four-month stay in this facility. It's like a logbook and I read it over now and weep for my poor, sad self.

My two most common topics of conversation, according to this book, are despair at being constantly moved (illusion) and my distress at the noise levels (reality). Rehab is not a place

I would call 'stroke-friendly', as strange as that may seem. In a stroke ward everyone knows the importance of quiet for people recovering from brain injury. By contrast, rehab is noisy, incredibly noisy and it distresses me greatly.

As the fog of psychosis lifts, following an increase in anti-depressants and the anti-psychotic medication provided by the psychiatrist brought in by my family, I become more aware of what's really going on and find myself somewhere on the continuum between extreme gratitude and total despair. I know I've been given my life back by people with extraordinary expertise. I know that my family's intervention has been selfless, constant and loving.

But now, clear-eyed, I can also see that I'm at the bottom of a mountain that I can't see to the top of. Survival is behind me, as is the quiet, stroke-specific world of the stroke ward, but I'm stranded between it and any semblance of normal life, trapped by total dependence on others. My therapy book attests to many tearful moments but also a strengthening — albeit fragile — resolve to find my way back and handle this new world.

I'd been told, within days of my surgery, about the paralysis on my left side. I was vaguely aware of it in the emergency ward, but now it comes as a real shock. In fact, I don't really believe it. It's only when I return to reality with a clearer mind that I start to believe what I'm told. In November I 'half-heartedly' accept that my paralysis has been there from the start, according to Petrina. Understanding that I'm paralysed on one side and have what is called 'left side neglect' is reality with a thump. These conditions are not going to be easily triumphed over.

Hemiplegia, paralysis of one side of the body, is common after stroke, affecting the opposite side of the body to the brain hemisphere affected by the stroke. As my stroke occurred in the right hemisphere of my brain, I'm affected on the left. That's why I continually slide to the right side of my bed and hoists are needed to move me about.

'Left side neglect' means a failure to attend to stimuli or objects on that side. It typically occurs following damage to the right parietal lobe. While hemiplegia affects my motor abilities, left-side neglect is more of a cognitive loss. Patients suffering 'neglect' need to be reminded to scan their dinner plate or the room around them, by slowly turning their head side to side. Only by doing this can they establish what exists on the neglect side. Essentially, I don't know that I have a left side to my body and I'm unaware of anything occurring on that side. I scarcely even know that side of my world exists.

Hemiplegia and left-side neglect are two distinct phenomena but they can occur together. Because my bleed was so severe, affecting both my frontal lobe motor cortex and the right parietal lobe, I have both. That presents many challenges.

I have to be reminded that there is a world on my left, so my family members all sit on that side to force my brain to awaken. I hear them saying constantly, in Kath and Kim style, 'look at me, look at me.' They also massage the left side of my body. Sometimes, lying in bed, I throw the blanket back and find an arm lying across my stomach and yelp in astonishment. Who on earth does it belong to? Who's in bed with me? When I figure it out, it makes me laugh.

But left side neglect is probably the most serious legacy of my stroke. I will never be safe on my own until I can overcome it. I can't even start to balance while it's there, as I lean so far to the right that I fall over. Even years after the stroke, I occasionally remove the clothing on the right hand side of my body but forget the left, or only read the right hand side of a menu, or injure myself if something is placed unexpectedly on my left.

Along with my visitors and therapists, I also put entries into my therapy book. My first one shows that I have some way to go with my handwriting, but my goals are clear. I'm starting to be Kathleen again, to think like Kathleen and I want the things that Kathleen values back in my life. With every day that passes, I feel more like Kathleen.

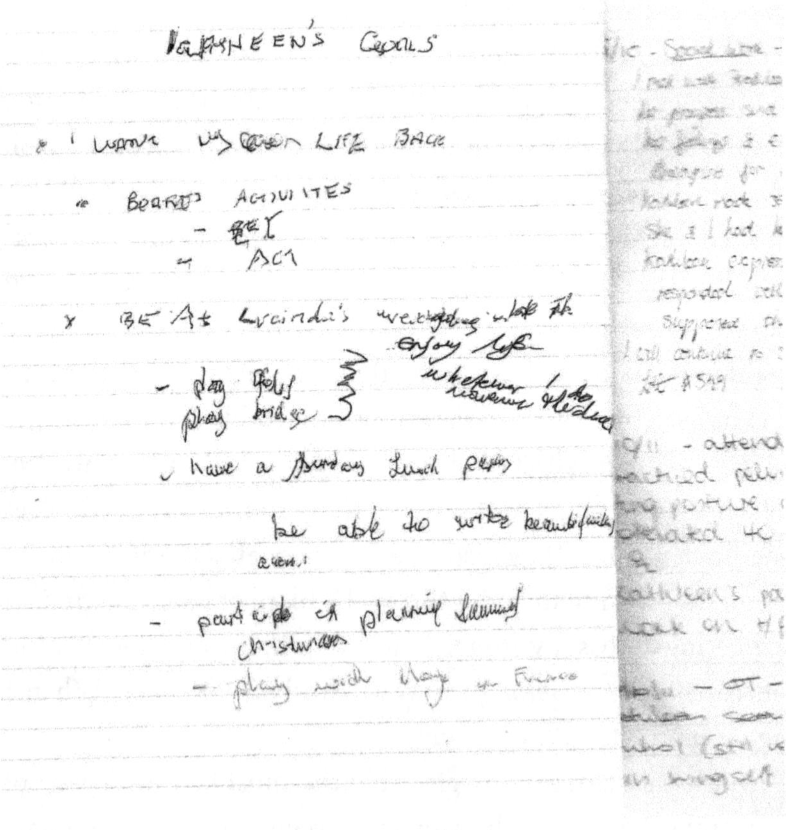

- *I want my life back*
- *Board membership/activities. Bionics Institute and FAST*
- *Be at Lucinda's wedding*
- *Enjoy life whatever I do*
- *Play golf*
- *Play bridge*
- *Have a Sunday lunch party*
- *Be able to write beautifully*
- *Participate in planning family Christmas*
- *Play with Moya in France*

Family advocacy in fast-stream rehab

There was this weekly pressure
— she's going to be sent out this week.
Lucinda

Staff said, 'nobody else has family like yours.'
Kathleen

Just as my family feared, my arrival in the fast stream (sub-acute) rehab facility, battling paranoia, confusion, depression, insomnia and fatigue placed me in jeopardy. In the short space of time since my stroke, they'd had to learn a lot about bureaucracy and, above all, about the need to fight. Their fear was that my previous psychosis had used up precious time and created a situation where my outlook was downgraded for reasons unrelated to my true ability to recover.

The threat hanging over me was that if I didn't improve within the expected time frame, I could be moved to the only option available, a geriatric rehabilitation ward. The thought of a geriatric community where only minimal recovery would be aimed for, essentially a nursing home in the aged care system, chilled me and it chilled my family. But there is a great demand for beds in fast-stream rehab. If I wasn't making any sense or showing obvious benefit, someone else might. The funding only allowed for six weeks at this level of rehabilitation, the level most heavily invested in recovery. What we all feared was my being 'written off', discarded or sidelined into the slow drift of geriatric care.

One day it actually started to happen. A young resident, deciding to be efficient and get people moved out of the ward, activated my discharge without any consultation with me or with my family. I rang Lucinda in alarm. 'If Lucinda hadn't been on the end of the phone, if Kathleen hadn't been able to phone and say, "I'm about to be taken to a geriatric unit", the outcome would have been very different,' my sister recalls. 'And I honestly believe that if we'd just let the hospital do it, Kathleen would not have recovered as well as she has.'

One of the main problems with the rehab model (at the time I experienced it) was that it wasn't designed for people like me. Essentially I was heading back to life from a situation that few survive. But in rehab, I was surrounded by people who'd just had their hip or knee replaced. Or they had been in an accident which they were receiving therapy for. They would be in and out of there quickly (hence the six weeks of funding). My needs were completely different. Due to the severity of my stroke, I needed *a lot* more rehabilitation.

Ideally, I would have joined a rehab system designed for people with serious acquired brain injury. I'm delighted to say that such a system does now exist in Melbourne, where people who have suffered traumatic brain injury are no longer subjected to terms such as 'slow or fast stream' but can enter a more tailored programme which acknowledges that their recovery may take longer, allowing them time to participate and recover according to their goals and potential for recovery.

To extend my stay, my family had to argue strongly that my

first few (psychotic) weeks hadn't counted because I'd been unable to participate in their programmes.

On two more occasions, they had to advocate for an extension to the original six weeks in rehab. Other threats arrived almost without warning, including a planned room change and then a decision to discharge me into a slow stream rehabilitation unit. Each happened without appropriate notice or the preparation time needed for a successful transition.

The hospital's position was that most recovery occurs in the first three months. At the eight week mark, my strengths were few and my weaknesses many. They used this argument against keeping me but my family knew by now that 'recovery after a stroke can occur usefully for much longer than three months.' I was in the unusual situation of having a slow recovery ahead, along with a high personal expectation of recovery, or at least the ability to lead a normal life one day. My family chose not to compromise my prospects of that recovery by bending to a system that wasn't designed to cater for me. The only path left for them was to fight until I could advocate for myself.

Despite numerous moments on the brink and several times having to suddenly gather and mobilise on site to prevent measures being taken, my amazing family prevailed. Instead of six weeks, I stayed at this first rehab unit for nearly four months, from October 2011 to February 2012. But there was never a time when they felt secure. My tenure was always up for negotiation. Without their active involvement, standing up for me through numerous meetings, I doubt I would be telling this story.

How much easier it would have been if the system could have taken into account my particular needs and allowed me to stay, without the destabilising threats. 'If we could have known she could stay at rehab, without the constant threat of a nursing home, which was so frightening, it would have taken all the pressure off,' says Lucinda. 'If we'd known she had four months instead of just weeks, it would have made such a difference. Instead there was a weekly pressure... she's going to be out this week.'

There was a price to be paid for the unrelenting advocacy, as well as the daily visiting roster and the ongoing provision of practical and emotional support each day. My family was becoming war weary. From their first experience in the emergency ward when they were told I was considered NFR, they had to change their perceptions of the system and how a family should behave within it. They never expected to become my advocate. Like most people, they believed the medical system was a good one and everyone should be left to get on with their work. But their first meeting with the registrar had alerted them to the possibility that vigilance would be required, and from then on their defences were up. The default position became 'Why aren't they doing more?' For this I am very thankful.

It was often uncomfortable for them. They understood that people mostly did their best under difficult or under-resourced circumstances, but still they wrestled with what they saw. They could see that I was simply being processed in the normal way but had to ask themselves, what if that normal way was not to my benefit? What if I became lost in the system of 'normal ways' and, in the process, was inadvertently denied access to a treatment that could have made a difference?

My family knew that I was not the sort of person to have gone quietly through the process of admission to hospital. Had I been able to, I would have keenly advocated for myself.

'I think we would have been very hard to deal with as a family,' admits Petrina. 'We were so much in there and at them, wanting to know what was going on, wanting to be involved.'

Taking action and fighting for me was also a way for them to cope with the confusion and despair of those days. 'Those first three months were so dark, stressful and exhausting. We were trying to get our heads around the medical system. In the end, you do just feel that you need to be a patient advocate for your loved family member,' says Lucinda.

In addition to the major advocacy, there was a myriad of tiny daily events. My scalp became itchy and they found I had nits. A treatment roster showed that I was given Endone, a pain medication that also causes sleepiness at 10am. A heat pack brought in by a nurse was found to work brilliantly on my painful shoulder, so they wrote in my therapy book, asking the nursing staff to please do it again if the pain persisted.

Continence remained an ongoing issue. Getting to the toilet took a long time and required effort from the nurses, especially when I still required a hoist to get up. My family learnt that I was often told by nurses to use a bedpan instead. But this would never help me, which was so critical. One family member wrote in my therapy book: 'Yesterday evening a nurse had been cross [with Kathleen] that she had asked to use the toilet again,' so they pleaded with the nurses to be patient, reminding them what an important step continence was for me.

Observation was another of the key gifts they gave me. Noticing, for instance, that my mental state deteriorated when the shunt was clamped off came from observing behavioural changes that were perhaps too small for the nurses. As I was mostly mute at that time, the variability *was* small. But nonetheless, it was there. The surgeon, visiting once or twice daily, would not have had the opportunity to see the effects of the clamping.

Observation of my early psychosis and subsequent action is another example. Observation doesn't require medical training, just the closeness of a loved one and the confidence to speak up.

Many meetings were held between my family and medical staff. They involved almost everyone except me. My family wanted me there but found that my presence introduced another set of problems. 'One of the first meetings we brought Kathleen into,' says my neuropsychologist sister, 'we had to contain her because she could go off track in her conversation, which would demonstrate what's called "lack of insight", a term often used about people with frontal lobe impairment who often say or do inappropriate things. Kathleen would talk about what she was going to do and wanted to do, which would feed into the treating team's perception of her as brain damaged and lacking insight, which could have fuelled the argument that she could be shunted off.

'In those early family meetings, when we did bring Kathleen along, there was a sense that we needed to protect her from herself. What's really needed is a balance, a way to differentiate between lack of insight and the need to maintain hope. But without a doubt, definitely, I think she needed to be in the meeting, just a little bit protected.'

Excerpts from Kathleen's therapy book:

October 27 2011

Kathleen is still having episodes of confused thoughts (this evening and last night). Stated that she was walking today, *still convinced she's moved to a new room etc. Please ask M re the antipsychotics and to check antidepressant meds are appropriate. Had 1$^{1/4}$ hours in chair in garden.*

Kathleen's brother-in-law, Mark

October 28, 2011

Kathleen's appetite seemed improved. Ate reasonable lunch. Turning to the left also improved. My friend is sad, which is quite understandable.

Jennifer P, Friend

November 11, 2011

Very tearful and upset this evening, saying 'for the first time in my life I feel like I don't want to live.' Talking pessimistically about her future. Feels her life is over. Concerned about her next step in rehab, where she will go. Was able to shift her perspective a bit with encouragement and support.

Petrina

December 12, 2011

Kathleen was brighter and very thoughtful. Although she remains fragile (understandably) in relation to thoughts/fears about her future, grief for the past and the impact of her stroke on her family (particularly her daughters), Kathleen is trying to find her way forward.

Psychologist

The burden of noise

As I've said, fast-stream rehab units are not really set up for people recovering from major stroke. Like most, this unit was full of patients learning to walk again after knee or hip replacements and young people recovering from injury and accidents. As a result, it was a busy, often noisy place, inappropriate for someone who has just had a massive haemorrhagic stroke and brain surgery. The recovering brain needs quiet and rest. Sleep is the time it assimilates the lessons learnt, in the exhausting process of making new connections and learning to function as part of a balanced and working body.

My first, shared room was opposite the kitchen/dining area. I was bewildered by the noise echoing in from the dining room and the large TV screen and people speaking loudly over it. My visitors frequently commented on this in my therapy notebook. My psychologist wrote, 'Kathleen feels the "inane and banal" TV is ruining her brain.' It was more than noise, it was a burden adding to my ongoing mental and physical fatigue, which was already so severe it was cutting short some therapy sessions and reducing the effectiveness of others.

Neuro-anatomist and stroke survivor, Jill Bolte Taylor, in her book *My Stroke of Insight,* describes trying to recover, desperate for silence and 'minimal sensory perception,' while the other patient in her room talks and watches TV. 'The TV noise from her half of the room was a painful suction of my energy. I considered it totally counterintuitive to my idea of what I found to be conducive for healing.' This brain specialist from Harvard Medical School describes sleep as a 'filing time for the brain,' allowing it to rest, file new knowledge away and protect itself amidst life's constant bombardments. She writes of the need to honour the healing power of sleep, interspersed with learning periods. 'I firmly believe that if I had been placed in a conventional rehabilitation centre where I was forced to stay awake with a TV in my face, alert on Ritalin and subject to rehab on someone else's schedule, I would have chosen to zone out more and try less.'

Agitation about noise brought another worry. Agitated people can't learn. Just at the moment I needed to progress, I was being deprived of the circumstances necessary for progress and recovery. 'Kathleen was the acquired brain injury person amidst people with hip replacements,' says Lucinda. 'We knew what the recovering brain needed in terms of quiet, so we became stressed about the level of noise she was living with. It's just not set up for people who've been so sick. We tried to make it more peaceful and the main TV was switched off at eight or nine at night.'

Christine Durham, in her book, *Doing up Button,* writes of the despair she suffered as a result of noise; snoring patients, doctors and nurses talking, vacuum cleaners, constant TV and radio, banging and crashing. She recalls, 'After two weeks of pain, noise, confusion and the bustle of the ward I felt I was about to go insane. I begged Ted [her husband] constantly to try to get me transferred to another hospital where there was a single room, or to the empty single room next door... I wanted that empty room more than anything I'd ever wanted.' Neither her husband nor the nursing staff truly understood her desperate need for silence and solitude, mistakenly thinking that companionship would be better for her. In her desperation, she would leave her room to sit near the lift well or in other quieter places, rather than her own bed. Eventually, in desperation, she locked herself in the bathroom until her needs were heard. Finally, in a room of her own, she writes 'settled in my room of silence, I could start to mend.'

Eventually, like Christine, I get a blessed room of my own, away from the noisy dining room, situated at the far end of a corridor. Its windows look out through tree branches to the sky. This is the room I referred to as my 'penthouse'. Its quiet, peaceful ambience and natural light through the trees have an immediate effect on my state of mind. I start to kick some goals in rehab.

Little things, like having control over my door, whether it was open or closed, gave me my first sense of control over my environment. I could surround myself with calm. When my family talked to me, I could concentrate on what they said. When Richard downloaded my favourite music onto an iPod for me, I could listen, rather than use it to block out other sounds.

When I returned to this unit a few years later (to visit, not stay) I noticed a strange contraption on the wall behind the main reception desk, a bit like a traffic light with a green light (happy face) and a red light (sad face). Its purpose, I was told, was specifically to raise awareness of noise levels. In deference to their brain injury patients, whose need for silence was now more appreciated, the unit aimed to ensure that its noise levels stayed in the green 'happy' level.

Changing energies

After a lifetime of independence, bringing up my daughters, working for a living, moving continents when necessary, the reality of being entirely dependent upon others was hard. It elevated the role of nurses and carers, and the effects of their personality. My day was greatly influenced by who they were.

Some brought with them a calm peaceful presence, sharing much needed laughter and welcome companionship. When they left I felt lighter and more hopeful even though they may have pushed me along quite mercilessly. Others were impatient and self-absorbed, not noticing my struggle. They left me feeling depleted and exhausted. Like the prisoner I was, I dreaded the change of shifts and what it would bring. I knew who I hoped would walk through the door who I desperately hoped would not.

I had spent my entire adult life working with people, helping them raise their level of self-awareness, so they can then relate to themselves and others more effectively. So it's a particular form of punishment to be lying on a bed, totally at the mercy of another person. Before my stroke, I could invariably solve personality issues. That was my speciality. As I describe, these are skills I bring to my situation later, but in these early fragile days, the personalities of the nurses loomed large.

I don't recall, in my pre-stroke life, ever being treated like an imbecile. Post-stroke, it was entirely different. Some staff seemed to think I was mentally deficient just because my responses were slower and some even spoke to me as if I was quite senile. I'm sure this is an experience common to all people with acquired brain injury.

A new experience for me in rehab is that of failing tasks, something that I hadn't often done in my pre-stroke life. Failure took some getting used to. Christine Durham similarly found that while rehab gave her hope for the future, there was a cost. For someone who had always sailed through tests, failing at some was a whole new emotional ordeal. At times she felt that trying at rehab didn't even make sense because the tasks seemed insurmountable. She describes looking at the other people struggling to achieve what appeared to be unrealistic dreams and wondering if she too was trapped in a similar cycle in a system that didn't seem to make sense.

I did find small places of respite, as one must. In rehab, that was a small internal courtyard, its blue walls and pots of hardy plants like cacti imparting a slightly Mexican feel. Sitting out in the courtyard was my first real taste of nature and fresh air. Retreating into this space with the sun on my skin made me feel that I'd almost escaped. I took my friends there, where we could sit away from the institutional life around us. But first I had to get out through the door. This was a big glass door that couldn't be opened by someone in a wheelchair. So when I wanted to go out, I had to wait beside it for someone to let me out, a bit like the family dog. When I wanted to come back in, I did the same, hoping that someone would spot me out there.

When I returned years later, I was really pleased to notice that a self-opening door has been installed, wide enough to fit a wheelchair. People no longer have to wait, like the family pet.

Friends arrive

As a companion, you're really unprepared for the various steps along the way, how long it's going to be and all the things that need to be done.

Liz, Kathleen's friend

When I'm no longer raving nonsense, it's time for friends to visit. Some older friends like Liz have already been, but she finds the sight of me in rehab, propped up in a gigantic motorised chair and still at that stage unable to speak, even more shocking than her first visit to intensive care. She describes me taking everything in, responding with my eyes but no more. 'I think that was the biggest shock for me because you think that she'll be in intensive care and then the next step is, she'll be out. You're not prepared for how long it is going to be, and all the stages there are — and some of them downhill.'

I credit so much of my recovery to the care, visits, phone calls and emails from friends. I cannot imagine how I would have fared without these wonderful people. In rehab, they become my second family: their flowers and cards fill my room and their support helps me through the long haul of recovery.

But what's supportive for me is often confronting for them. In the past, we've shared lunches, wines and good times but the truth is that I'm no longer the good company that I was.

Friendship means something quite different now. It can be hard work and sometimes guilt replaces the laughter of the past. My joyfulness has gone. Our mutual spontaneity is not there and, like all stroke patients, I can be difficult company at times; self-obsessed, depressed and poor at acknowledging another's pain.

So my friends withhold their own stories and shape their conversations thoughtfully, not wanting to burden me with their problems. Or they hold back on telling me some of their more exciting news, aware that there may be things I don't want to hear. It makes for a lopsided friendship. I know they mourn for me and what has been lost between us. These are the moments that have to be negotiated with patience, out of love for friendship past and belief in friendship future.

My situation inevitably brings out emotions in friends that may relate to past events in their own life or fears about their future. Seeing how I look and how reduced my life has become can be confronting. Some find seeing evidence of the devastation life can bring to be far from easy.

My counsellor, Pam, explains, 'Kathleen was a very organised, energetic and able client. I found myself wondering how something like this can happen to someone like that. Why Kathleen and not me or someone else? It can be hard to empathise with what she has been through when a part of me doesn't want to know, doesn't want to face the fact that life can be so cruelly random and fickle. It raises the inescapable fact that 'I am now in that age group where events are less able to be relegated to those that can be tut-tutted away as awful, but distant and only ever happening to others.'

During her visits she senses the adjustments, a sort of changing of gears that takes place between the past and a new future.

She describes seeing both me, and also another version of me, all at once. 'Her smile — that was the first thing I saw — was just the same as ever, it seemed to me. But on embracing her, I became acutely aware of the wheelchair, now representing her immobility. Noticing her left arm supported on a pillow — now a rebellious, unresponsive part of her body, and her leg, similarly needing to be put in its place each time it strayed without permission — I felt a small shock all over again at the reality of this stroke, and the havoc it had wreaked on such a good brain, a good soul.'

Another friend, Kate, a trained nurse, finds me lying on the floor in a state of agitation. A male nurse kneeling beside me is holding my hand, comforting and trying to calm me down. As Kate enters, he looks up and says, 'Oh look, Kathleen, here's a friend' and I amaze Kate by immediately apologising to her. She had been due to stay at my house while on business in Melbourne and I must have remembered that my stroke had prevented that. If she feels relieved, and thinks everything is normal, it doesn't last long. Within minutes, I am again agitated, thinking someone has stolen my wallet. For a few moments we manage to achieve a quite intimate connection but when my sister arrives and talks me through my agitation, Kate feels immense relief. 'It was utterly confronting for me to walk in to that, my dear friend. She has beautiful hair and there she was, with half her hair gone and in this confused state. I came away thinking, "This is horrific and there is a massive journey ahead for my dear friend, and I don't know how this journey is going to go."'

Michelle, a friend who is also the managing partner in a legal firm that was a client of mine, visits at about the same time and is also confronted by the sight of me lying on a bed on the floor.

Like Kate, she leaves thinking that I will be unlikely to recover my life.

My friend Jennifer describes her pain at seeing 'such a beautiful woman in such a predicament.' To her it must have been an even more acute shock, as we had played bridge together just the night before the stroke. I had even texted her the next morning — all very routine and normal. But within hours of that, she received Lucinda's 'devastating' text.

'After Kathleen's stroke the family kept us informed and we received some very helpful emails and text messages, but there came a point when I realised that I had to stop making enquiries. They had enough on their plate and needed some space. I think by the time Kathleen did get visitors, she was wanting to see people from the outside world. My mother had had Alzheimer's so I was used to hearing people make inappropriate comments, so that part didn't faze me. Most of the time she made total sense, but every now and then she'd say something and you'd just know it couldn't possibly be true. But why would you think it would be different to that anyway?'

Jennifer brings what she learnt of brain impairment from her mother to our new friendship. 'I can remember, when I finally realised my mother didn't have a hearing problem but wasn't processing information, that I was able to be a lot more gentle and understanding. It's a passage and it's quite difficult at times.'

Another friend, recovering from her own significant catastrophes of 2011, hesitated when she heard my news. She was grateful for the emails from my family, but didn't feel up to visiting. 'How could I face her and her catastrophe when I was so engrossed in my own? Time passed and I was reassured by her survival and progress but still I had not been to see her.'

She describes the turmoil that many feel in her situation. 'The longer I waited the harder I was finding it. What would she look like? Would she still be the elegant and beautiful woman I so enjoyed and respected? How could I face another example of life's seemingly arbitrary lottery of pain and suffering? What would I say?'

When she does visit me in rehab, she finds herself ashamed of her 'self-absorption' and her fears of what she might find. 'Kathleen welcomed me, her determination to overcome and succeed evidenced by the cards, instructions for movement and inspirational messages pasted over the walls of her otherwise stark and depressing room.'

Guilt is a frequent partner for my friends. Have I visited enough? Done enough? What *is* enough? Knowing the long days I endure, dependent on everyone else to function, some feel survivor guilt, or just guilt at feeling relief when they return to normal life after a visit. Recognising this, another friend, Alice, wrote, 'Thank you Kathleen for always welcoming me when I visited and for not judging me when I didn't.'

Each dear friend brings a valuable gift of herself and some put in enormous effort over a very long time. This is the great value of friends. Each understands a different part of you. I urge anyone visiting a friend who has suffered something like a stroke to bring with them something that expresses the value of their friendship. Maybe it's doing their nails (which my friends did) or bringing some music or flowers. As Liz says, 'It does sort out true friends. How much are you prepared to be involved, how much can you cope with, seeing a friend distressed?'

The friend who had hesitated, burdened with her own very considerable problems, brought me a painting from her artist daughter. In rich red colours, it features three words: *Never Give*

Up. I hang it on my wall immediately and it hangs on my bedroom wall today. Jennifer and Alice visit together and, sensing that I want some entertaining and news from the world outside, cheer me up with tales of the silly things everyone has been doing. Jennifer says, 'She wanted to hear something other than medical things. Alice and I intuitively knew that was our role. I wasn't going to enter into what might be or what might have been, or the future. My role as friend was entertainment and distraction and she just had to get through it one day at a time.'

I laugh with them, but my depression is also evident. They understand. Who wouldn't be depressed? But when I speak of loss and grief, as I do often, they wait an appropriate amount of time and change the conversation. They also encouraged me to work as hard as I could. 'When she had to use the slide, we'd push her along, saying come on, come on.'

Alice's gift is a mantra that we share over the phone, something that gives us words for those moments when it's hard to connect over distance. Called Sa Ta Na Ma, this primal mantra is recited in conjunction with finger movements, pressing a finger one at a time on the thumb, one hand at a time. Sa means birth and evokes the sensation of emotion and expansiveness, Ta means life and creates a feeling of transformation and strength, Na means death and stimulates universal love and Ma means rebirth and evokes the quality of communicativeness. This mantra is both consoling and simple to concentrate on when thoughts are scattering. It is a lovely and helpful gift.

Many friends work to protect my dignity, just as my family does. It becomes important to them that I look good, having always been so careful about my presentation. Jennifer says, 'Family are so busy on so much, they may not see if your hair is straggly or you've got five hairs coming out of your chin. That's what friends are for. You think, "There but for the grace of God go I."' So they paint my nails and ensure that the 'girly' part of my life isn't extinguished because of what has happened. They bring 'champagne' (cider) which we drink in flutes, and sushi and play card games, making sure I have whatever 'little pleasures' they can provide. They ensure that even if my left hand sits at an awkward angle, my nails are painted a lovely colour. They shave my legs so they look and feel smooth.

Even my hair becomes a topic of conversation and concern. Some like the slightly gamin look that the short haircut, necessitated by having my hair shorn for surgery, has given me. Others, like Lucinda, miss my thick, dark hair. I regrow it. It's an important decision. I need to retain my self-esteem and confidence if I'm to put my energy into recovery. My looks should not be collateral damage and part of the valued positivity that friends bring is their demonstration of love, which they manifest in caring for my appearance and my confidence.

The cards and flowers that people send are enormously important. It doesn't take much imagination to understand what it must mean for a person staring at the wall from the vantage point of bed, if the walls are covered in heartfelt loving messages. These cards become my most meaningful possessions, something defiantly 'Kathleen' in my otherwise entirely institutionalised life. I guard them jealously and stare at them for hours. It's no accident that in my moments of psychosis, it's these precious objects that I fear are being stolen. They are all I have! During that time, my long suffering brother-in-law, Mark, was frequently called upon to count them for me (he recalls there were over 100) to satisfy me that they are really all there. I might have been confused and psychotic, but I knew these were the last remnants of my sense of self when so much else had gone.

When I look at the cards, it's as if I can hear the people saying, 'You are still Kathleen, you are loved, we are thinking of you, not everything has changed.' Even after the visits and emails begin, the cards remain a tangible gift. In my confusion and exhaustion, I may forget friends' visits, but their missives are always there, their influence persisting through days of endless boredom and even psychosis.

In *My Stroke of Insight,* neuro-anatomist Jill Bolte Taylor, who suffered a left hemisphere stroke in 1996, called her mail 'a touching reinforcement of who I was before the stroke.' Collecting it, looking at pictures and reading messages made her feel surrounded by love, and long after her recovery she remains grateful to those who reached out to her in that time and believed in her.

Progress — standing up!

What we take for granted, getting in and out of a car,
on and off the bed, on and off the toilet seat,
all had to be painstakingly relearned.
Alice — friend of Kathleen

Rehab is about training the brain to deal with the body in different ways. On arrival, I had poor initiation, severe left side weakness and left side neglect, over-activity of muscles and an impaired sense of where my limbs were or where my body is in space (proprioception). In essence, I was immobile, almost completely unable to move. Hoists were required to move me about, I lay in a tilted chair and slept in a bed on the floor because of the constant sliding to the right.

For me, as for many other stroke patients, left side neglect will be the most serious and ongoing problem, along with the fatigue that makes everything difficult. Despite its centrality to all my problems, my neuropsychologist sister was concerned to notice that left side neglect increasingly became a side issue within the therapy of the occupational and physical therapists. 'No-one was owning, overseeing or co-ordinating the management of Kathleen's left side neglect. And some of the work being done was misguided.'

They would like the involvement of a neuropsychologist. An earlier assessment at the eight-week mark of the important 12 week post-stroke interval, which described me as having many weaknesses and few strengths, was not followed up. When they enquire, my family is told that while neuropsychologists are allowed to conduct tests, this particular rehab centre (unlike many) doesn't use them in cognitive rehabilitation therapy. This role is divided between speech therapists for language and reading, and occupational therapists for functional therapy.

But a major turning point occurs with the lifting of my psychosis: functional progress starts to happen quite quickly. With a clearer head, my involvement in therapy increases. I started learning to sit up without support, which is when I began to regain continence. I was expected to be performing transfers (moving from bed to chair for instance using slide boards) at around six months, but after several weeks I'm transferring on a slide without needing the assistance of a hoist. In my therapy book, a physio who had seen me earlier returns to visit and writes, 'I was amazed at how good you were with a slide board transfer after only a couple of weeks!'

When I arrived in rehab, I was unable to stand by myself. Even if I held on to a railing, I still required support from two others. Lucinda recalls asking a nurse if I would ever be able to stand up and hold on to something by myself — it seemed such a distant goal. She was assured that I'd be able to stand up by myself in a month or two, and that is what I did. When, with the assistance of a hoist, I stand for the first time since my stroke, I almost pass out with dizziness. But it felt like incredible progress.

Learning to stand and walk is a massive ordeal. At the gym, my first task is to sit and be balanced amidst cushions. Learning to stand requires a hoist initially, and later a walk between parallel bars. At every stage of balance, stand and walk, my left side neglect creates huge difficulties. It makes balance seem impossible. Even though intellectually I know that the centre of my body runs down from the top of my head, past my nose to my navel etc., the actuality is very different. I overcompensate to the right, and overbalance. It's very, very hard. I am filled with fear — everything around me feels like a big open space where I'm precariously positioned, because I just don't know where my body is in that space.

Sixteen weeks post-stroke I start using an electric wheelchair, which is part of the therapy to develop left hand scanning and awareness of where the body is in space. I quickly discover that a wheelchair is both a new level of mobility and a new liability. Unable to recognise *what* my left is, let alone what might be lurking there, I take off without having scanned the environment — or having checked the speed on the dial — and repeatedly injure myself. My sister suggests that the occupational therapist writes up a four point 'take off' checklist and puts it under the control stick, to help me remember what I have to do before taking off.

There are days when I feel confident as I drive around, certain that I've overcome my left side neglect, only to drive straight into an obstacle. I end up with bruises all over my left leg, some very scuffed doorways and feeling greatly discouraged. It forces me to realise that I am not as advanced as I thought I was. It is all, basically, trial and error, often too much error, but slowly I get to the stage where I can manage.

As I drive, I grimly repeat a little mantra, 'left right, left right', to remind myself to scan from left to middle right. But I gradually become more competent and the chair allows some fun and laughter as I compete in wheelchair races against my grandson, Asher, on his scooter along the path outside. And the zoo, which is just down the road, suddenly becomes accessible as Emma takes on the big task of leading her three children and me in a wheelchair single file along the road. We go several times and suddenly I'm a grandmother again having everyday fun with my grandchildren.

As Christmas approaches and progress finally becomes evident, my family start to feel some joy amid their exhaustion. It's been a gruelling three months. While I write shaky Christmas cards to friends, my daughters plan a special Christmas, one that will take an enormous amount of organisation. We are going (they hope) to share our post-stroke Christmas lunch inside the place I have missed unceasingly since my stroke, my beloved home.

Christmas

It was bliss to be in my own home and
with my family, and out of rehab.
Kathleen

My house was my refuge from the world, situated in a quiet street in a leafy inner suburb of Melbourne. Every part of it had been designed to be place of peace, with large windows and changing elevations overlooking my tranquil garden. It was my home in every sense of the word, a reflection of my inner self, a place of light, air and nature, often filled with fragrant food and the sound of opera.

Lucinda and Emma are determined not only that I'll spend my first post-stroke Christmas day there but that I'll also sleep the night there, along with them and their families. Initially, it seemed a mad dream, almost impossible to realise, but slowly it materialises into reality. Long ramps are organised to get my wheelchair up into the house, and Richard gets his tool kit to make a tiny ramp for a pesky step that may cause a problem. A hospital bed is hired and put in the living room, so I can sleep downstairs, as well as a special toilet seat and a chair so I can sit at the dining table.

To have my two daughters work so hard to do this for me! And it was a *lot* of work. As I watched them working, I thought back, as I so often did, to Lucinda's birth, three years and nine months after Emma's. Here I was, about to give birth again and wondering if I could possibly love this new baby with the intensity I loved Emma. We mothers love so intensely — how can such intensity double itself to admit another? I wasn't the first to wonder if it could happen!

But when this tiny baby was placed in my arms, I remember whispering, 'Hello Lucinda May' and experiencing a rush of love surge through my whole body — a love which grew daily. Emma quickly assumed the role of a wonderful big sister. My two gorgeous girls, who remained loving friends. When they were little, one of their favourite books was a delightful story called *Big Sister, Little Sister.* The three of us knew it simply as 'Here Blow.' It refers to a moment when the little sister is crying and the big sister holds out her handkerchief. 'Here blow' she says gently. Every time we looked at it, we all knew it was really Emma and Lucinda on those pages.

To attend the Christmas lunch, I needed to reach a certain degree of mobility. One of the nurses said he would show me how to get out of bed without hoists and how to stand holding a pole, so that chairs can be swapped behind me. He pledges to have me ready for Christmas, so the girls can achieve their goal. They are delighted. 'We thought she would always require a hoist to get out of bed, and be in nappies and such,' says Lucinda.

So on Christmas Day we all ate lunch together, then took my beloved grandchildren to the park we used to visit. 'It was so lovely to have her there, to lunch with Emma and I and our families,' says Lucinda. As planned, we stay the night, all of us together.

But the joy of sharing Christmas, of being still alive and — briefly — in my own home, is overshadowed the next day by my return to rehab. 'Putting her into a maxi-cab the next day and back to rehab, that was terrible, one of the most heart breaking moments of mum's recovery,' says Lucinda.

For me, it was also a goodbye. That was the last time I would ever be in the home I loved so much. I farewelled my garden, knowing in my heart that this would probably be the last time I saw it. Christmas with everyone was very special, but it also showed how dependent I was on others. I feared, as did my family, the imminent move out of fast to slow stream rehab. I needed every bit of rehabilitation I could get.

The long stay in slow-stream rehab

February 2012 – June 2013

She made her room her haven, with postcards and flowers and music and paintings but the centre drained her spirit. The air hung slowly, devoid of movement. I sensed the sadness in her voice and I felt sad too.

Alice (friend of Kathleen)

Eventually, in spite of my family's extraordinary and successful efforts to prolong my stay, I must move out of the sub-acute unit (fast stream rehab). I am extremely reluctant to leave my room with its views of trees and sky. I dread the move. I worry that the next step in the process, slow-stream rehab, will be a step down in my rehabilitation prospects, as indeed it is. It's a place where the ability to stay for longer is counter-balanced by the reduced amount of rehab on offer — and by reduced expectations of ever returning home to live independently. Most people, when they leave slow stream rehab, are destined to live out their days in a facility such as an aged care home.

The actual move is easy. I don't have far to go. The long-term rehab unit is situated just a few metres down the road. I'm taken there by one of my favourite nurses, David. As I make my way along the path in my wheelchair, he walks beside me, chatting and pushing a hospital bed piled high with my belongings!

My new home is a one story unit built in the early 2000s. It's bleak on the outside, low and institutional. Inside, the long corridors are gloomy and oppressive. It could scarcely look less welcoming, or feel less like my new 'home'. When I think back on this place, I see there were many positives, but the negatives still give me nightmares.

Both rehab units are part of Royal Melbourne Hospital's expansive Royal Park Campus, set on the edge of the Royal Park parklands, just beyond the city centre. The campus has a mix of buildings, from a 19th century hospital through to modern centres, set amidst curving roads and patches of garden. At the edge of the campus, amidst the parkland, a golf course abuts the main carpark. To those who have to live on the campus, the occasional shout of a golfer and whack of the ball provide a reassuring sound of normality and a sense that the outside world still exists. Often, on the long, slow hours of a rehab weekend, I sit and watch the golfers walking the course — a rather sad entertainment, separated as we are by an immense cyclone wire fence and the even greater distance of my wheelchair bound disability. Watching them reminds me of the many days I spent golfing with my friends, then sharing lunch, laughter and companionship.

I stayed in slow stream rehab for 16 months, in which time a series of events occurred in my own family that made the campus, its buildings, even the golf course area, feel like a place of grief. As if the strain of my own situation was not enough for us all, death and illnesses will send us reeling again.

Years later I was to return to this campus, to visit specialists. Just the sight of it filled me with sadness and grief, leaving me almost numb with despair. Eventually I realised that returning to a place that was literally imbued with grief was not in my best interests and went elsewhere, hopefully never to return. Sometimes aspects of the past have to be consigned to the past and not revisited.

On arrival, I was given a private room inside the unit, due to my family's extensive intervention (meetings had taken place before I arrived). When you are confined to a room, it is your world. The first room had a view into a courtyard, the second — joy of joys — to the outside world where I can see trees and a pathway along which people walk between buildings. I watch them all day long, so unthinkingly free in their movement, out in the sun, enjoying fresh air and daylight, or scurrying along in the rain. How I envy them!

Like the blue courtyard in my previous rehab unit, nature provides a balm for my soul as I slowly recover. It's not just nice to have, it's way more than that. I NEED this, to see the sky, trees, grass, birds and people. Are we not animals? Why wouldn't access to nature be part of our recovery when our world is upended? The greater the distance from my stroke, the more strongly nature's beneficial influence calls to me.

When I arrived in this unit, 24 weeks after my stroke, my family had been told plainly, 'She will move and this is what we have to offer you.' Although they are unhappy that I'm going to slow-stream rehab, it is undeniably better than a geriatric unit, which is the alternative. Like them, I find the whole concept of 'slow to recover' (in fact, slow anything) absolute anathema! My entire psyche is focused on getting well as quickly as I can. Now I want as much therapy as I can possibly get and I find myself feeling quite resentful when other people, probably because of their own brain injuries, refuse to go to physio. It feels like a wasted session that I could have had.

No longer trusting that my needs will be met or my desire to become independent will be honoured, my family had meetings with the managers of the unit beforehand. They were assured that I would get a private room (which happened) and receive the same intensity of rehab that I had been receiving (not the case). In the meeting they work hard for concessions and guarantees, trying to do so without antagonising the people they will be dealing with in the near future. After their meetings, we sit down for a coffee and agree that what they have negotiated and agreed to 'seems pretty good... an outcome we can live with.'

But the first battle soon arrives. It turns out that the unit has a policy of not providing any rehab for the first month. This is to allow patients to settle in and probably works well for most, but it's a disaster for me. I'm in the early post-stroke months that are so important to recovery and there isn't time to waste — enough of that was done during my psychotic interlude! It simply reflects the gap between my needs and the needs of those around me.

Most of my fellow patients in slow stream rehab will, when they leave this unit, go to a geriatric unit — irrespective of their age — or live in community assisted housing. A more fortunate few, who have tenure from a previous funding model, will stay here indefinitely. They are not ever expected to develop sufficient self-reliance to go home, which is precisely what I am determined to achieve. I don't know where home will be — my lovely house, with its many steps, is looking increasingly remote — but from my first day here neither I, nor my family, entertain the possibility of my being in care for life. I will come home.

As time goes by, my therapy hours dwindle. My family is told that I have had my share of rehab. Some family members also wonder if I'm not contributing to the slowing pace, if the long months of dependence have made me slightly institutionalised. They notice that I'm no longer setting new objectives for recovery. That as the rehab I receive is reduced there is a corresponding reduction in my personal energy and commitment. They call the National Stroke Foundation to see what they should do. The advice they receive is what they already know so well; 'The more rehab the better, the more hours of physiotherapy the better, the more occupational therapy the better. You need to fight for her.'

Of course, they've been fighting for so long, and will continue to fight until I leave, just short of two years after my stroke. But they try again and look at bringing their own private therapists in. Staying within the system, they felt as though 'After a while, we were banging our heads against the wall,' says Petrina.

Life inside

The time in here is often an easier journey for those who are not aware of what is happening to them.
Nurse at the long-term rehab facility

Sixteen months is a long time. I spend it in an enclosed, internal world. This is surely the hardest part, the loss of ordinary living and experience. The weekends are worst, and long weekends without rehab are excruciating. Sometimes I feel that I am rotting away, just fed and watered like a cat whose owners are on holiday. The visits of family and friends are what I live for.

The long corridors of the facility are purposely dim because of the brain injury patients, but it makes the unit feel even more isolated from the world. The staff tries to break its grim bureaucratic feel, enlivening walls with bright decorations, colourful words and pictures: small tokens of the human spirit asserting itself against bleakness. But it retains a subterranean feel, a confronting place filled with the sights and sounds of patients who are suffering very severe and intractable brain injuries.

In one room, a man lies on the mattress on the floor, groaning and calling out. Another man, his head deeply scarred, lies quietly while his wife sits alongside, day after day. A handsome teenage boy, slumped to one side in his wheelchair, has his keyboard on his lap, his mother and brother patiently learning the new world of communication. In the TV room, rows of patients line up in their wheelchairs. My heart goes out to these people and their families. Unless you are a healthcare worker, who eventually becomes inured to their working environment, it feels like a place of despair.

As my friend Kate observed, visiting was 'Hellishly confronting. You don't expect to see a dear friend there. I'd seen some pretty awful sights but these were confronting — young people who'd addled their brains with drugs.'

'Some of the people there couldn't communicate, were awake screaming at night and the walls were paper thin,' my friend Liz recalls. My neighbour in the room next door, a young mother, brain affected by addiction, attacks me when I ask her to switch her TV down late at night. The staff attempt adjudication, but our competing needs are a problem. Each patient has rights, and my neighbour's rights to have TV blaring at 2am need to be considered.

Strangely, I am again the 'odd one out' but for different reasons. 'There was a difference between her and the others and the severity of their head injuries was part of that,' Mark recalls. 'She was a duck out of water.' Cognitively, I am fine, but I'm trapped inside a body that I can't manage, which I can barely control. I am my body's prisoner, confined to my institutional room because of this heavy, unyielding thing that refuses to obey me.

I tried to make my room my haven. My friend Kate describes how relieved she was to see it within this confronting environment. 'The place smelt awful, but then you went into Kathleen's room and it would smell like Kathleen, beautiful perfume and there were always flowers, her motivational things up on the wall and surrounded by cards. She always managed to be beautifully groomed when I arrived. She would ask me to help, maybe with a shawl or to trim the flowers, and it felt good to help. As often as she could, we'd go to the rose garden or under a tree. She hosted me, which she's so good at. Or we'd go to the coffee shop and she'd buy me a coffee. She did her best to normalise her life and our friendship.'

Trips away are wonderful, but there is the inevitable return to this institutional world. My wheelchair is a massively heavy contraption that means I have to take maxi-cabs, which are heavily booked and can't be trusted to arrive on time. I have spent so many anxious hours waiting, and having to ring and ring to make sure I am on their list. Each doctor's appointment involves long waits for the taxi and I become anxious, uncertain if they will arrive on time, or even at all, and unable to help myself in any way.

Once inside the taxi, I sit propped high up like a puppet in my wheelchair, swaying nauseatingly around every corner. Some of the drivers are kind. Others have to be cautioned that if they don't slow down I'll end up vomiting inside their cab. To use normal taxis means that I have to take my folding chair, as my wheelchair can't fit into a normal car. In that case I'm entirely dependent upon the drivers to push me out to the cab and then push me where I need to go at the end of the journey. It's not a courtesy that you can rely on. With no understanding of my immobility, they often react poorly to the situation.

One day a driver wheeled me out of his taxi and into the hospital vestibule and simply left me there, facing a wall. Fortunately before I had to endure the indignity of having to call out for help (hello? hello?), my friend Liz arrives. 'Are you enjoying the vista?' I hear her familiar voice behind me and feel relief flood over me. But the indignity and helplessness linger. 'We had a laugh about it,' says Liz, 'but that shocked and upset me even years later. Kathleen kept saying to me, "He left me here and I couldn't do anything about it!" I could list them, pages long, moments like that.'

When I return from visits to the outside world, or trips with my family, I feel despair creep over me as the car slowly edges its way through the familiar parklands towards the campus. I'm almost panic-stricken as the 'real' world disappears behind me.

But there are positive moments too. A nurse walks in and recognises me from the stroke unit, where she had nursed me. She can't believe my progress. She tells me, with great confidence, 'You will walk out of here!' From then on, I am determined to do just that. Like many of the nurses, she is marvellous and helps my recovery enormously. I owe them so much for their kindness and caring, not just to me but also to Lucinda. As always, there are one or two who are not so good, and one is so bad I ask for her to be kept away. I can't afford to lose the energy she takes.

In contrast, people like Emelia, my occupational therapist, were a great support. I looked forward to her visits. She was bright and fun and reminded me of Lucinda. Importantly, she acknowledged my determination to move beyond a rehab facility and matched it. Emelia recalls the time as being 'A horrible situation for Kathleen amidst the lack of resources and her own family tragedies. But Kathleen was amazing. She'd be upset but then, next day, ready to go again. Nothing could keep her down and that made me keep fighting for her.'

The rose garden

It is impossible to describe my life at this facility without mention of the rose garden. It's a most surprising find, almost directly across the road from my unit; an entire 19th century formal rose garden, complete with geometrically laid gravel paths and low box hedges, all leading to a large central fountain.

This treasure is a relic of the campus's earliest days. It is situated within a large courtyard that is surrounded on three sides by the double storey barracks-style wings of the old hospital, now neglected and covered in peeling white paint. Once an actual army barracks, then a refuge for the destitute, a poor house and later a hospital for the elderly, the building was once home to Melbourne's infirm. Some arrived as small children and lived their entire lives here.

I can't wander the paths of the rose garden, which are too difficult for my wheelchair, but I can sit in the courtyard on the old, cracked bitumen, and stare in. The ghost of patients past can be felt. One can almost see them sitting through long afternoons in their wheelchairs under the verandas, staring into the rose garden or walking slowly through the narrow parterre paths among the roses. In winter, the spiky branches of the rosebushes add to the old courtyard's funereal atmosphere, but in summer their colourful blooms mitigate the feeling of sadness and neglect, bringing welcome life. The flowers are a reminder of the power of regeneration.

Although there are other, sunnier, lawns and trees around

— which I make good use of for family get-togethers — this old rose garden in the cracked bitumen courtyard is my special place to sit with friends, or be alone with my thoughts. *This is my life now. This is what my choices have contracted to. How do I manage what has been given to me?*

Family sadness and new tragedy

Outside the rehab unit, during my long months of recovery, the process of life and death continues, as it must.

Within months of each other, both my parents die. I can see these two wonderful people towards the end, bent over their walkers, with loving smiles and whispered cuddles, telling me, 'You are very much loved. You are the bravest person I know.' When, years later, I read Jill Bolte Taylor describing her mother coming to hospital, slipping under the sheets, into the bed and wrapping her arms around her stricken daughter, tears prick at my eyes. We are always their children.

Knowing my love of flowers, my mother had sent them to me regularly. They had both visited me at every stage of my recovery. As a family we celebrated their 65th anniversary with a picnic on the lawn near my rehab facility. As their oldest child, I have always felt especially close to them. In the summer after my stroke, my family had needed to move them into care. They were fiercely independent and lived in their own home until the age of 88, but Dad's infirmities had become too much for Mum to manage. She wouldn't let him go into care without her, so they went together.

While my sisters and brothers-in-law are wonderful, as the eldest of the five daughters I would have been expected to pull my weight. I am sad that I cannot help with the packing up of their home or settling them into their new one. Family members and friends take me to see them there, so I'm able to enjoy visits, but I feel as if I have added to their burden.

Mum dies in October 2012. She had been in palliative care and she dies with all of us, her beloved family, beside her. Someone takes a beautiful photograph of Dad holding her hand, which he does for hours until she dies.

Returning to rehab afterwards is hideous. My sisters come into my room, joining with me to plan the funeral and together we create a beautiful and moving ceremony. But alone in my institutional room, I think how much my own house and environment would have soothed me. But the nurses and kitchen staff surround me with kindness and thoughtful actions. I think back on them every day with gratitude.

We all rally around Dad, who is stoic as always, but we know he is grieving terribly. We had planned a party for their joint 90th birthday, and he tells us to go ahead with it.

He dies just a few months later, in February 2013, in the Epworth Hospital. I take the call from inside the rehab unit. Petrina was with me and we reflected on what a blessing it was that we were together. With Petrina and Gordon, we go to say our final farewells. Again I return to the bleak surrounds of the unit and find myself surrounded by kindness from the nurses and the wonderful women in the kitchen, in particular Wendy and Kerry.

Between my mother's death in October and my father's the following February, the family does share a happy event: the marriage of Lucinda to Richard in November. My father even manages to come along to the service and we are all filled with joy that he can see this happy pointer to the future.

Christmas 2012, the second after my stroke, is quite different to the first. We celebrate at a house owned by the brother of my son-in-law, Emma's husband, Piet. Much less equipment is needed for me, which is a good thing, and I stay two nights instead of one, which is even better. The joy of being out of the rehabilitation unit and with family is immense, and Christmas, like Lucinda's marriage, stands out as a light happy moment in a time of continuing sadness.

Soon after her wedding, Lucinda receives a diagnosis that shocks us all: breast cancer. My constant, tireless advocate is now facing her own battle and I, her mother, am helpless to provide any assistance. When I talk about grief later in the book, it's this loss that I think of most. To have a daughter who needs your help and be unable to provide it is a tragedy for both of us. My grief and despair feel overwhelming.

At about this time I find myself in a bureaucratic vice — the bed I occupy is evidently part of a funding model that only lasts a certain amount of time. My family is told I no longer warrant it and that new patients require it. We learn that only nursing home beds are long term, which we had not known.

The complexity of funding models is a whole new world of unknowns. Hidden walls appear which have their origin in pages of legislation we know nothing of. We learn one set of funding guidelines and then find we are actually under the aegis of another. It's a never-ending learning curve. Some of the staff members are not happy that I've come to the end of my funding, but it's not the first time they've seen it. For my family and me, it created huge anxiety about what would happen after my discharge. Where would I go? What would it cost? Would I only be eligible for aged care? Did everyone fight so hard for two years, just to finally see me languish in an aged care facility? Could I get an aged care package that would pay for what I needed to live outside its walls?

While I was in rehab, Lucinda and Richard had come up with a plan for me to live with them when I finally left. They had been working on their house, extending their property to give it a spacious hallway and doorways wide enough to fit my wheelchair. But that is now unthinkable. Lucinda is not well enough to take me. She needs quiet and rest as she embarks on a year of surgery, chemotherapy and radiation.

I also won't be returning to my old house, and never will. With its lovely changes of floor levels and many steps, it's no place for my wheelchair bound reality. Digesting that takes its own time and I allow myself to gradually accept what I already know.

In the end I didn't walk out of the unit, as the nurse had predicted, but the nurses did form a guard of honour and I remember it with gratitude. Used to the disappointing reality of watching their patients depart to a lifetime of care, I sensed their genuine pleasure to see someone leave for a proper family home. The fact that I didn't actually walk out doesn't seem important. That will come and her words gave me great hope at a time I needed it most.

In that nearly 16 months of great change and sadness, both my parents died, their last sight of me no longer their vibrant daughter, the one who could solve anything, but a woman condemned to living her days in a rehabilitation unit. Then my beloved daughter Lucinda became unwell. After looking after me for so long, she now needed the care that only a mother can give, and I was locked away. I felt I had failed her and my parents, by being unable to give either the support I desperately wanted to provide.

June 2013

A tiss and a tuddle: home at last

Finally, the day I had repeatedly been told would never arrive arrives.

I go home, to a real home, far removed from the world of institutions. As Lucinda focuses on her health, my sister Petrina and her husband Gordon have stepped up with an incredibly generous offer. They have a single bedroom unit at the back of their house, along one side of their back garden. Although occupied by a friend of theirs, they decide that this place, just metres from their back door, could be made to work for me. Obviously their friend needs time to move, so Gordon also suggests that I spend a few weeks in intensive rehabilitation at a private inner city hospital. It's an inspired idea. I have a wonderful time receiving more rehab in a day than I'd been getting in a week at the slow stream rehab unit and it prepares me wonderfully for the move, lifting me out of the torpor that had descended on me.

It also reduces my fears for the great test I'm entering. Can I cope on my own? What if I fall? Will it work? Independence has been the aim since I first realised I'd had a stroke, but faced with the reality, I am naturally fearful.

But even the word 'home' sounds so good. I say it over and over and it relaxes me, as though I'm headed for a utopia. In a way, I am. Having a welcoming and nurturing home is one of my key passions, a defining characteristic of what makes me Kathleen. Denied this key part of my personality for so long, I think about it a lot while I juggle the fear and the excitement of leaving for independence.

Again, my wonderful family gets busy on my behalf. My brother-in-law, John, builds a wide, sturdy ramp leading up from Petrina and Gordon's garden to the unit's front door — a ramp that I use every day and which gives me freedom to move without needing anyone's help. Other family members visit my house and pack what I'll want, including paintings and favourite objects, my desk and computer, and my tubs of azaleas and gardenias. The unit may not be home as I knew it, but it's filled with things I love.

And joy of joy, in my bedroom, my bed. Not a hospital bed, but my own proper queen-size bed, the sort of bed an adult sleeps in. On my first night I lie in it, feeling really happy. A huge moon slowly makes its way over the sky and the garden glows with soft, natural light. It feels miraculous.

My little niece, four years old when I move into her back garden, embodies everything about this world of home and family when she knocks on my door to announce that she has come for a tiss and a tuddle. Now that she's older, it's a kiss and a cuddle. Imagine how it feels to be in the bosom of a loving family after years of linoleum corridors, strangers and institutionalisation.

I love to hear the children playing and watch them bounce on the trampoline. Even their occasional bickering brings a smile. Normality feels and sounds so good. I look forward to my Sunday invitations to pancakes and coffee, just down the ramp and into their house. I have dinner with them some nights and am happy when I can bring some of my home-made soups, prepared in my kitchen. Oh, the taste of my own food.

Outside my window, their chickens Isabella and Mabel and the two rabbits Oscar and Basil (collectively known as the chabbits) share a lovely enclosure that takes up much of the yard; they unknowingly become part of my recovery. It's laugh aloud funny to watch Oscar, who has an excess of attitude for any rabbit, round up any chook who dares go near his food. Our local blackbird family frolics in the birdbath and every morning their beautiful singing is the first thing I hear. From my kitchen window I see trees and sunlight.

When, on almost exactly the third anniversary of my stroke, a fox slides into the garden and silently kills the chabbits, we cry like children. The two hens and two rabbits are buried together, laid gently on a bed of straw and covered with flowers. Petrina collects Mabel and Isabella's last eggs, hardens them in the microwave and the children place them gently beside their bodies. They write a lovely message on a stone, which is placed on top of the grave. There is not a dry eye around. I cry, thinking how much I will miss their antics and that my hours sitting in my recliner and looking out to their compound will never be the same. I thank them for the laughter they brought and the sense of energy and renewal their little lives gave to my own slowly recovering life.

In time we find new inhabitants for the chabbit enclosure, starting with Ash and Cotton, two rabbit siblings. Rabbits and chooks are part of our family and life together, although Ash's acquired nickname of Houdini doesn't auger well for his future.

Strangely, one of the best parts of being 'home' occurs when I go away. Getting out from the rehab unit was always difficult. I felt so cut off from the world that I was almost disorientated in it. I could go to a lunch with friends, but felt like a stranger in this busy, doing things world. Much worse was the moment I came back to my room, like a prisoner returned to their cell. Especially after a weekend at my daughter's house, to return was dread indeed. Now, it's quite different. I go out with friends, we have fun and I go home just like anyone else. No dread.

Part of this lies in the ability to create one's own environment. The 'welcoming and nurturing home' that is such a part of me finds expression when I can invite friends to lunch and make them welcome. They don't have to perch in sterile rooms feeling uncomfortable, or we don't have to escape to the rose garden to find solitude. I did my best at the rehab unit with cards and positive messages everywhere — nurses and dinner ladies always said my room had a lovely feel about it — but it didn't feel like home. Being at home is nurturing for my soul in a way that being in an institution could never be. I've come to accept that 'home' is a unit in my sister's back garden and even see my good fortune in it. My sister comments, 'There is no way, pre-stroke, that Kathleen would have entertained the idea of living in a granny flat in Petrina's back garden, but she's done it with good grace, taken it on the chin. As someone so proud and independent, she would never, ever have seen her life being this way.'

One morning, I wake pre-dawn to find moonlight streaming in my bedroom window. Soon after, the blackbirds start their dawn chorus. I feel so happy and think of the moonlight that used to stream into my house through its huge, high windows. Suddenly I realise what is so obvious; moonlight and blackbirds are everywhere and, in that moment, I let go some of the longing I feel for my old home.

I feel proud to be here and feel that I've made a big step. The next step is to leave this unit and live on my own, in a house I own. Meanwhile I have learnt to accept that this is the new me and to feel some satisfaction that, after all the dire predictions, I've fooled the buggers. I also have to accept that there may be limits to where this will end. But this is an excellent stepping-stone to living independently and to a semblance of my old life. I know it will be different, but it will be a good life full of love, laughter, meaning and purpose.

Paying the price — the cost of advocacy

We really got the sense over that two years that we were 'the difficult' family. I remember saying to a family member at one stage, I feel like we are in One Flew Over the Cuckoo's Nest *— not in 2012 Melbourne!*

Lucinda 2014

There is a price to be paid for everything, even acts of kindness. My family paid with exhaustion, stress, guilt and illness. It seems so unfair that I have cost them this while they stepped in to save me so many times.

I cannot help but worry that Lucinda's illness, arriving just as I turned the corner towards independence, had its origins in the stress of that time. For close to two years she worried about me, about how I could be best cared for, as well as bearing the burden of daily oversight and being involved in many, often difficult, advocacy meetings. How could I not wonder? Christine Durham's son was diagnosed with diabetes after her car accident and she also questioned the role of stress in his condition.

Petrina, who tends to deal with the upsets and tragedies of her life in the way of medical people, by being calm and doing what needs doing, recalls that sometimes she and my other sisters would just look at each other and ask, 'Are we in a nightmare?'

When I went into the stroke ward, Petrina came down with shingles, that classic opportunist illness in times of stress. As she says, 'I'm sure it was my body saying this is not OK. We were in a nightmare and it was responding to the stress.'

Another sister describes the slow, wearing effects of the 'driving, the hours at the hospital, taking our parents to visit, lack of sleep due to anxiety about Kathleen.' It all began to take its toll. Survival guilt crept in and she wondered how she could carry on with her own life and enjoy herself. 'A wise friend pointed out that I had no choice but to lead my own life and to let go of some control, that Kathleen would be well looked after. However, it would be a long time before I could stop thinking constantly about her.'

My family found the change between the early days and the slow stages of recovery was another part of the journey they needed to adapt to. 'In the early stages it was keep doing, get on with it, fight, support, all high energy stuff. But one of the hardest stages for me was when Kathleen plateaued out during long term rehab. There was tremendous guilt that we could walk away, leaving her there — all we could do was support her, take her out and do things but at the end, it was back to the unit. It was hideous leaving her there.'

The constant meetings with medical staff had been a massive source of stress, coping with conflicting information, pushing for the best, living with the feeling that they were 'the difficult family.' Inside the family, there wasn't always agreement on how to go forward. Inevitable friction arose from a group of intelligent people thrown into a whirlwind like that. Everyone wanted the best for me, but there isn't one pathway labelled 'best'. You have to decide what that will be.

Moments of real dilemma inevitably arose, such as when

I entered the rehab system. I went into fast stream rehab initially because my family fought hard for that. But now, looking back, they sometimes wonder if maybe their hopes and mine outpaced my actual ability, for fast stream rehab left me exhausted. As ever, they had acted out of the understandable fear that I would be left languishing in a backwater, missing out on something valuable and perhaps, as a result, viewed as someone who might never recover.

Lucinda explains, 'Our worry was that she wasn't going to get the rehab she needed, that she would be missing out, so, there was lots of discussion and emails about that. But now, looking back, I would say any rehab she received would have been good. Probably her brain wasn't at the stage where she could process fast stream rehab and so perhaps starting with slow stream would have been better and it might have been easier for her if we'd just let it be. But we were so scared she'd get stuck there and never make it to fast stream rehabilitation.'

Some medical people had advocated that I should go straight to slow stream rehab. But my family were uncomfortably aware that their dismal predictions often precluded the possibility of what I *might* be able to do, given the chance. 'Despite the experts progressively claiming that Kathleen may never recover, may always be incontinent, may never walk again, may have suffered personality changes and may not be able to speak, we felt that her best chance for recovery lay in her receiving as much physiotherapy, occupational therapy and speech therapy as possible. That's why we felt that Kathleen should go straight from hospital into fast stream rehabilitation — to maximise her recovery.'

We are all united in the belief that, despite these moments of questioning, what they did was critical to my recovery. My nursing trained sister is adamant about the role of family support: 'It was essential, from attending meetings for Kathleen's care to advocating for her needs and negotiating over her rehabilitation requirements.'

My friends, who observed my family's efforts, without exception believe that it was instrumental in my progress. Liz says, 'I am absolutely certain that without that voice and advocacy, Kathleen wouldn't be where she is now. Lucinda was almost her mother's voice. Everyone needs an advocate and maybe one is better than half a dozen.' As she points out, having a relative in hospital is a high stakes situation, where the difference between action and no-action can be someone's life. 'There's no point thinking, later on, I wish we'd done this or I wish we'd asked these questions.'

Kate makes the point that advocacy has the potential to 'Wake people up to what is possible. This is what I saw Kathleen's family do and it was essential.' Kate went through a similar experience when her partner was seriously ill, spending many hours advocating for him and talking on the phone, making things happen. 'Inevitably you can make yourself unpopular and the potential downside is that you or the family member can be punished. But I tried to be as friendly and polite as possible, while also being strong and assertive.'

Liz wondered about the potential downside of making me unpopular when I moved into slow stream rehabilitation. 'I felt that in slow-stream rehab there was a loss of dignity and less compassion. Sessions would be cancelled, staff complained that because she was vegetarian she was demanding. It got to the point where I really thought twice about bringing anything to their notice because once you walked outside they might take it out on Kathleen with little things, like making her wait for a shower.'

It all really opened my eyes to the fact that no matter how intelligent you think you are, how comfortable you think you are, when something like this happens you are completely helpless and it's hard to know who to turn to. Who do you liaise with? Who is the central person? Who mediates? I watched Kathleen sitting there, helpless and dependent, with critical physio appointments cancelled without warning, a wheelchair that was dangerous taking weeks for someone to even look at, follow up visits from various medical staff delayed till next week or the week after, someone meant to liaise with someone else and never getting around to it. The lack of coherence and follow-up was shocking. Kathleen's family advocacy was critical and they were extremely effective.'

My friend and client, Michelle, compares it to her own medical turning point, after a diagnosis of a blood clot in her leg. Increasingly exasperated with the lack of information given to her, she reached the point of thinking, 'I needed to understand what they were doing to me and why, and not just be *told what to do.*' Eventually she said to the doctor, 'This is *my* body, this is *my* life and these are *my* questions!' From that moment on, she found everything changed. 'I was no longer just a person with a blood clot. Kathleen needed to do what I did, but obviously she was unable to, so Lucinda and her other family did it for her. They were amazing.'

Was there another way?

Lucinda was showing her love, care and support for Kathleen. She was able to advocate for her mum and still maintain her role as a daughter. She did it so well; maintaining her professionalism and not getting drawn down by unfair systems. She was inspirational.

Emelia Young, Occupational Therapist, slow stream rehab

Looking back, three years after the stroke, Lucinda sometimes wondered to what extent their advocacy was also, in some respects, their own way of dealing with the situation. She occasionally wondered if the outcome would have been the same if they'd stood back a bit and let the process go forward. But her conclusion is always the same; that their advocacy made an important difference. Every other family member and friend agrees with her and some believe it made *the* difference.

'In the end,' Lucinda says, 'you react in the way you know how to for loved ones, in the best way you can for them. The medical staff were always telling us it was going to be a long journey and would take time, but it doesn't make sense at the time. We were always thinking, "Yes we know that, but we want to know more about what is happening NOW." At each point, we needed to know. That is just how it is.'

Emma agrees, 'We always felt the bar was set very low on her recovery prospects, so our constant advocacy was to counter the fact that people seemed to have these low hopes for her.' Petrina believes in stressing the importance of letting staff know who I was, and how determined a person I was. 'Telling the staff about Kathleen, telling them that she wanted to have her life back, did stimulate some of the people we spoke to. If we hadn't told them, how would they know?'

It makes me wonder what happens for the patients who have no one to fight for them, people who don't have family. The system does allow for a state appointed advocate, which is a worthy step. But as the nurses know, family and friends are the critical people. An appointed advocate can watch a patient and ensure they don't get lost in the system. They can make sure their rights are upheld, but, of necessity, it's an administrative function. Without the impetus of love, and without knowing the person as they were before, the advocate's role is to ensure that a reasonable level of care is maintained. But someone in my position needs people who will fight unceasingly to get the absolute best, defying predictions and the grimmest of prognoses along the way. That takes love.

The return on the family's hard work and advocacy is their knowledge that it made a difference. It was worthwhile, even though looking back, there is a sense that I had entered a huge 'post-stroke machine' which could not be diverted. What they did was affect things along the way as I progressed through the system.

They have an undeniable sense of pride that I got through. Increasingly, we are having laughter and conversations as we did before the stroke, and the mutual caring that has always characterised my family has been proven under the direst of situations. My wins are theirs and they have demonstrated the power of 'never saying never.' The rest is up to me.

First realities

In the early days of living in my unit, I have a transitional care programme organised by the occupational therapists I had been working with. Being assessed as 'very high dependency' means that carers visit me twice daily and with their level of care I begin to relax. I can do this. The reality is that for the moment I need a lot of help to live independently and couldn't manage without them.

The funding system again is critical. My 'transitional care' package lasts 12 weeks. Other packages are available but when we apply, we are told it could take 18 months to reach the top of the waiting list. So, naturally, during that first 12 weeks of transitional care, Lucinda and Emma worry incessantly. What will happen when it runs out?

These are the realities of funding packages and bureaucracy for people in my situation. To add complete stupidity to the equation, I find I can't apply for funding until I actually need it: the wait may be up to 18 months. When I apply for a wheelchair this happens and by the time one arrives, the hiring cost may have added up to be almost as much as the chair. I ended up buying one but that's not an option for many people.

The funding problem is the first real problem I solve by myself, and I feel proud of what I do. Firstly, I think it through as if it was a business problem, of the sort I had been handling two years before. It felt a bit like the start of life again. I decide to use the 12 weeks (which finally extended to cover 18 weeks) of the transitional package as an opportunity to ring as many funding bodies as possible, to get that critical long-term package I must have.

Each agency I speak to that is responsible for funding says the same thing. I need to wait. But, with my business hat firmly on, I know that each conversation has the power to lead me to another — if I ask. And that's what I do. I ask everyone I speak to, who else do they think I should call? I ask for a name. Finally, someone suggests the name of an agency and tells me that the government has just released some new packages. This is exactly what I'm waiting to hear. Within days my new funding is in place, exactly in time as the transitional funding package runs out.

This is luck, but only of sorts. It is also determination and self-advocacy, just as I had used in business and just as my family had used for me. It pays off. There is always a way, but you have to push for it. Sometimes it can be as simple as realising that a person has inadvertently given you inaccurate information regarding your entitlements or funding. We tend to believe what people say. But I find, for instance, contrary to what I've been told, that I can access a carer when I visit Emma in the country. This brings a whole new level of freedom. I also learn that my funding can be transferred when I move house, which I had been told wasn't possible. I learn more and more and find, if I budget carefully, I can access what I need and my package will be mine for life. I particularly appreciate the 'escort services' (their wording!), which mean someone comes to take me shopping, to appointments and out on activities — which really contributes to an increased sense of wellbeing and the possibility that life is returning to normal.

So I have learned to question constantly. What one person tells you isn't always true, as well intentioned as they may be, and funding is subject to change. It's an important issue. We are reliant upon funding, just as we are reliant upon carers to help us up in the morning and into bed at night.

With independence comes control — at least over some things. I now have some input into who will be my carer, something I obviously couldn't do in rehab. When a person walks into your room, takes you into the shower, helps you put your clothes on, prepares your lunch and later in the day returns to help you into bed, it's a matter of self-respect to have a voice in who that person is. Most carers are extraordinary and committed people who love their jobs and get joy from helping people. I've met some remarkable women and shared some great laughs. But, as ever, there are a few who should have chosen another career. In that case, I have the power to request a change. It's as though I'm now a grown-up, granted some say in my life.

Preparing food is an overlooked part of normal life. I have fresh fruit and vegetables delivered to my door and, with help from my carers who do the chopping, can make simple dishes to eat and share with others. It is a joy beyond words when my daughter visits me and I serve her delicious, nourishing soup from my own kitchen — I feel like a functional mother again.

But independence brings its problems, inevitably. I fall several times, especially in the early days but even years later. The real issue is not to lose confidence afterwards. I have three falls soon after getting home and make use of the security mCareWatch I wear, which allows me to call any of three people on a contact list with just one press. Help arrives immediately, but I feel bruised, in limb and emotionally. Much later, I survive a weekend on my own without Petrina and her family — which is a landmark — and then, later, after four whole days on my own, I fall during a physio session. Feeling pretty pleased with my progress and regained independence, I had become a bit over-confident. I end up shaken and in pain, but with nothing broken. I go on.

Having me home is a release of tension for my family. They hated leaving me in long-term rehab, hated feeling that there was nothing more they could do, and bore the guilt of walking away after each visit while they got on with their lives. When Petrina and Gordon take me to live in their little unit, everyone is profoundly grateful to them. Together as a family, they have found a way through every situation.

The idea versus the reality of coming home takes adjustment for all of us. It raises difficult questions of what I have to accept and what I have to keep pushing for. And for the family too, it has meant moving to a different place in acceptance. Petrina says, 'We've all interacted with that dance between positivity and acceptance in different ways. Kathleen needs care, but she's not in a nursing home and she can do a lot, so she's defied that centre of gravity. So the family too has had to move from advocacy and fighting — all that active, high-energy stuff — through to "the system is there for us... we don't need to fight it, we need to use it." It's acceptance.'

I'm now in charge of my future in a way that hasn't been the case for over two years. It was two years that both changed me completely, and not at all. But my past has keys to my future. What I learnt and practised as a businesswoman in my previous existence can now come to my aid, I hope. Tentatively, I start practising what I preached all those years ago.

PART II

The Emotional Journey of Recovery

The great thing in this world is not so much where we stand as in what direction we are moving.
Oliver Wendell Holmes

Home — now what?

Finally making it home raised many questions, as of course it must. There were so many steps to go. The question was, what direction should those steps be in? I needed to aim for a future, but what would it look like? How could I best embark on the next level of recovery?

Stroke — like much traumatic injury — is really all about recovery. From the moment medical expertise has saved your physical life, it's all about what you do to recover. It's really an inversion of other diseases which affect your body progressively over time, but remarkably similar to other major life events which bowl you over out of the blue: loss of a loved one, loss of work, and all the other major and massive disruptions that life can serve up which throw you off your normal life trajectory. These are the events that force you to change, and fast.

You go straight into recovery mode and you start swimming towards the shore. But quickly find the shore isn't where it used to be and no longer even looks much like what a shore should look like. You're aiming for an unrecognisable place, where you'll be building your future.

The only certainty is that you can't do anything about what's already happened. Everything is 'Now what?' The way you respond to that question is how your future will look.

During this time (and still today) I drew on strategies from my previous life, strategies that I had seen work for others. I had worked with many clever and talented people who fell short of their potential, often due to limitations in their thinking. They were, in a sense, handicapped, just as I was. These people were mostly lawyers, senior managers or directors. There was no sense telling them what to do; I had to bring them along with me.

I quickly found that, just like them, I'm not too good at being told what to do and so I needed to take a subtle approach even with myself!

I also thought about my assets, what I had going for me that I could use. It occurred to me that the immense goodwill of my friends was an asset — like an energy source that I could use, and I knew they wanted to help, to do something that would really benefit me. I needed to guide them, to create some strategies that would take this up from individual acts of kindness and goodwill to more enduring structures that really help long-term. We came up with some good strategies, some of which are still in use.

Being hospitalised for two years gave me plenty of time to reflect and see what worked for me and what didn't, what gave me strength and determination, and what sapped those critical attributes. I now needed to build an emotional response to my situation to create a scaffolding that would be a support. My thoughts had to become my ally and not another obstacle to overcome.

In this section of the book, I share what worked for me and I hope that some or all of it works for you. But I start with a section on facing facts. I think that before building positive strategies, facing the (often unpalatable) facts is necessary. Then you can start to plan a new life.

The debit ledger — anger, depression, grief, loss of self, fear … and medical predictions

You don't have to feel full of hope to behave in ways that challenge the grief. But you need to acknowledge it, and then quietly get on with action. Hope and despair can sit alongside each other. They are not opposites. You can be full of grief and also grateful and proud.

Pam Rycroft, Psychologist

We need to face our demons and call them for what they are, which is why I have lumped all the negatives together. I call them the debit ledger, perhaps because of my business background, but also because the debits tend to work together. Thinking of one tends to lead to thinking of them all. We all have debits in our lives that we have to work around and they force us to use our credits wisely and forcefully to get through.

Anyone who has suffered physical trauma like stroke receives a lot more physical than emotional rehabilitation. Emotional recovery (naturally) can only be attended to once we have made it to life, but it's a lonely world we emerge into, in which we sink or swim according to our thoughts. In front of us is the yawning abyss called 'Who am I and what am I doing?'

I arrived home wheelchair bound, unable to work, suffering relentless exhaustion and almost overwhelmed by what I'd lost. I was reliant upon carers to get me up in the morning and into bed at night, and almost everything else in between.

If I thought being home meant returning to Kathleen and her life again, I was wrong. The list of losses I'd suffered ran through my mind like a bad movie. My independence, my role as mother and grandmother, my business and the means to earn an income, my ability to just stand up and walk, go for a coffee, do anything at all without planning, needing people, waiting for others — in fact so many steps that I was exhausted before I began. This was not who I was.

But then who was I? I was no longer the successful professional I knew myself as. My business life closed overnight. I could no longer even attend board meetings; I had to resign 'for the moment' as the other board members kindly put it. My house, that citadel of 'me', was going to be sold. I had used it as my working space and it was the place where I had invested my whole identity.

A carer said to me at around that time, 'Gosh you've lost a lot, haven't you?' after she'd asked me what I used to do. Of course, the things I told her were just the start! I hadn't mentioned the lost time when I could have been seeing my children, my grandchildren, or travelling the world.

My ability to find love was severely compromised and with it went my dreams. On top of the loss, or maybe part of it, was the huge trauma of starting out again in my sixties while handling all this grief, loss, terror and bewilderment. The daily stresses have to be handled even while assimilating the post-traumatic stress. There was no sense denying them and trying to be happy. A debit ledger is normal. I had lost a lot.

Anyone facing this situation will find that losing their sense of identity to major trauma, and building a new one, is about as challenging as it gets.

I found this loss of self to be at the core. It was worst during the two years of hospitalisation but persisted when I got home. I was a mother who loved being a mother, a grandmother who loved being a grandmother. Yet the reality was, I was unable to help my daughters other than just 'being there.' Even in her illness I was unable to do anything for Lucinda. All through her treatment, I felt as if there was a big black cloud over me.

When my grandchildren came to visit I couldn't even hold them — and in the early days I didn't even see them, as they hadn't been brought in to the hospital. As Christine Durham, in her book, *Doing Up Buttons*, wrote so movingly, in her bleakest moments 'I have lost me.' At times of greatest depression and grief, she even asks if she is still a member of the human race. Jill Bolte Taylor, in her book, *My Stroke of Insight*, wrote, 'I had stepped beyond my perception of myself as an individual.' Her grieving started even as the first stroke symptoms arrived, which, as a neuro-anatomist, she quickly recognised for what it was. In that instant, she anticipated death and grieved for what she believed would be her lost life, and for the innocence that evaporated with the realisation that she was not invincible.

Durham says that if someone had explained that feelings such as loss of pleasure, emotional numbness, despair, anger, hopelessness, dazedness and why me? were normal for someone in her situation, in post-traumatic stress, she would not have experienced so much guilt and stress. She learns this only years after the accident. What she needed, she says, was a sufferer's manual, to help her through the grief of loss of being a mother, a wife, having freedom, a career and the ability to drive.

As I cast around for clues about how to create this new, unfathomed life, I found the ground beneath my feet was constantly eroding due to the dire predictions about my future. If I learnt anything during this time, it was that predictions are just that. They are not defining guidelines to the future, but simply based upon the experience of others. I am not others. For everyone who conforms to medical predictions, there are those who don't. I decided to continue being the person who doesn't.

If I had listened to the medicos from the word go I would have given up. It's that simple. I've defied the odds at every step. Doctors predict to the best of their ability and their abilities can be very great, but their predictions don't spell your future.

The 'don't get your hopes up' line they adopt comes from an understandable concern not to give false hope. But who knows the power of our determination? As we learn more about brain plasticity, we routinely exceed the wildest hopes of researchers only a few decades ago.

We used to believe that certain abilities, once lost, were lost forever. That the brain was like a car engine, but supplied without spare parts. So patients listening to their doctor's predictions were limited in their expectations and hence their recovery, simply by the state of knowledge that existed about the brain at that time. As we learnt more, more became possible in recovery. But the brain itself hadn't changed, just our knowledge. Our sights could expand to a wider expectation of the possible. And it's just the beginning, early days.

Jill Bolte Taylor explains this in her memoir. Although it took eight years for her to fully restore physical and mental function, her early knowledge about brain plasticity, as a neuro-anatomist, was fundamental. It provided her with a guide as to how to treat brain cells to help them recover, as well as a belief that they could. This was at a time when this knowledge was not widely known by others.

'I believe I have recovered completely because I had an advantage. As a trained neuro-anatomist, I believe in brain plasticity — its ability to repair, replace and retrain its neural circuitry. In addition, thanks to my academics, I had a roadmap to understanding how my brain cells needed to be treated in order for them to recover.'

In the previous chapters we've seen, from the first prognosis of being in the NFR category that, had the doctors' predictions been accepted as the only truth, I would probably be either dead or in a nursing home. Even the shocking post-operative headache I was told would be there for life went away. What a terrible thing, to be told to expect debilitating headaches for the rest of your time on earth!

It still goes on. The medico who was asked to prepare a report for the conciliation of my Workcover insurance claim wrote that I was a candidate for a nursing home for the rest of my life. As fate would have it, the week he wrote that report, I was actually having my first weekend entirely alone in my house. Petrina and her family went off for two days and I lived in my unit without family around. It was a huge step.

There's a line here between having delusions and having goals — but who knows where that line is? There are certainly some people, who, when they hear me list what I'm going to do in the future, believe that I'm demonstrating lack of insight. Essentially, that my damaged brain is giving rise to fanciful notions. As my neuropsychologist sister explains, 'That's so unhelpful. What it means typically is that you're brain damaged, but really what Kathleen is grappling with is this *huge change* in her life. It's a forever change, so why would she give up on all of her hopes on day one? She might say something aloud to test the waters, and who am I to say she won't do it? Kathleen knows the limits. She gave me her golf clubs but I would never say, "Kathleen, you'll never play golf again."'

Of course, some things do need to be accepted. I'll never be the same as I was before my stroke. I may never drive again (but I'm starting to think I might). I won't be playing golf anytime *soon,* or buying a new golden retriever… but I might in future. My family has been very good in understanding my need to maintain goals, while respectfully suggesting I may have exceeded reality when I do go too far.

'Kathleen might say that she's going to work again, and who am I to say "you're not?"' says my sister. 'She may well work again but in a different form. As a family, you don't dash hope. You might say, for instance, "Maybe you'll do this, but in a different form to before."'

Dealing with the debit ledger

We don't even know how strong we are until we are forced to bring that hidden strength forward. In times of tragedy, of war, of necessity, people do amazing things. The human capacity for survival and renewal is awesome.

Isabel Allende

Dealing with the debit ledger is not a one-man job. I engaged a counsellor to help me through and she suggested that I deal with the grief in whatever way possible, as I seemed to be holding a lot in. The grief we feel after this sort of trauma is not always publicly acknowledged. It's known as disenfranchised grief, part of the deal of what has happened to us and often quite invisible to others. How can I explain the grief I feel about not being able to help my daughter through her illness? That I will never again (probably) experience the everyday freedom of getting into a car and driving off? Even waiting for a carer to arrive is a form of grief. It's hidden away inside my experience. If I explain to someone that I feel this grief, they can understand but it may not have occurred to them.

My counsellor suggested having a good cry, talking about it and writing it down. This is what I wrote down:

I am grieving for my loss of independence. Being able to jump into a car and go wherever I please. I used to love driving to the west, to see my family in Western Victoria.

I miss regular contact with my daughters and my beloved grandchildren.

I miss being a support to my daughters. I grieved terribly that I could not help Lucinda in that ghastly year of treatment.

I grieve for my beautiful home. I hated selling it. It was just so perfect for all aspects of my life, family, professional and social.

I resent the intrusion into my home of carers day and night.

I grieve for my possessions in store and the fact that I haven't seen them for years.

I grieve dreadfully for my professional life. It was wonderful making a real difference in people's lives and that of their organisations. I loved my time in Sydney, Canberra, Darwin, Arizona, California, New Mexico, Hong Kong and Bahrain. I was in flow in my business and was thriving on all the activities, from dinners and meetings to forums.

When both my parents died, the grief was made worse because I was in rehab. I had grieved when they went into care and I couldn't help my sisters with the practicalities, sorting their home out etc. Missing them, and the finality of their deaths, was more than I could bear in the impersonality of a rehab unit.

Some time has passed since I started these notes. I think I must have processed a lot of grief, as it is now an ache rather than a torrent. There were days when tears remained close to the surface and my emotions were very labile. Even as I threw myself into therapy, my conviction about my own strength wavered. Could I really walk again? Would I ever be able to use my left hand? I kept these thoughts to a minimum, not wanting doubt to creep into my conviction that I'll return to a normal life.

Another counsellor suggested an image that I like to use — to imagine grief and hope like two aspects of a giant wave. As one rises, the other falls. They are connected, for without one we have less need of the other, but when the grief aspect rises we need to work hard to ensure we are not swamped. The hope side is the counterpoint, the connecting tension that will soon rise also.

Still fear creeps in. When I get a bit tired or het up, I start to feel like I did on the day of my stroke. Immediately fear sets in. Am I having another stroke? Sometimes I ask others if my face appears different, as I try to calm the terror inside. It's natural to fear another episode, especially when the first one seemed to appear out of the blue. It's part of the process of recovery to change your life to build physical wellbeing, to reduce that possibility. To handle the fear by putting in place positive action to reduce the risk factors.

Building emotional strength after stroke is not unlike building physical strength. You take it step by step. I wanted to walk quickly — in fact I wanted to walk out of rehab — but it was explained to me that goals of that magnitude needed to be broken down into smaller steps. In order to walk, I needed first to spend hours exercising the muscles of my left leg, to try to establish new neural pathways from my brain to my leg. It felt very strange to break the task of walking up into tiny bits. I would try to stand and, like an oversized toddler, fall backwards onto the bed. Sometimes my laughter at how ridiculous I felt would turn into tears of frustration.

So it is with emotional strength. You build little by little. You fall backwards at times but the goal remains and in small, incremental steps you develop the emotional strength that true recovery requires.

Jill Bolte Taylor, in *My Stroke of Insight,* described recovery as 'agony'. After her surgery, she asked herself if she was really prepared to put in the effort that recovery would require. She decided that the answer was yes, but that it was a decision she had to make and remake 'a million times a day.' Over the following years (it took her four years to regain a smooth walking gait), she visualised what it would be like to run up steps, keeping the circuitry in her brain alive until she could actually do it. Along the way, with each improvement, she thanked her brain for responding so well to her efforts, believing that making her body a happy place by her thoughts would induce 'some sort of vibration within my body that promotes a healing environment.'

It's a beautiful blend of determination and gratitude, of noticing the things that go right while keeping the main prize in steady focus. We are alone in our decision and the responsibility is entirely ours, but the acts of others can make a big difference. From the day I was allowed flowers in my room, something inside me changed. I felt locked away and out of sight, but I read the notes people wrote, saw their flowers and gained strength from their support.

The credit ledger

Success is walking from failure to failure
with no loss of enthusiasm.
Winston Churchill

The credit ledger, the upside to trauma (including our existing strengths prior to the trauma) is the energy source we use to build a future life, just as any credit ledger is the lifeblood of a business. It's also true that credits in life and in business tend to present themselves less conspicuously than debits! If we do take notice of them, they have enduring and profound strength, as the new research into what is now called 'post-traumatic growth' demonstrates. We'll look at that in more depth later, but, at its simplest, it means that when all else is swept away, we get to see what might have previously been hidden and gain valuable insights into life and how we can live and operate beyond the borders we'd previously set. Trauma opens our eyes, however reluctant we might be to do this. It can make us not just a different person, but a more insightful, humane and complete person, as a result of being forced to allow new things into our scope.

Jill Bolte Taylor found that a whole new world opened up to her as a result of her stroke mostly when she realised that her original 'I' had not survived the stroke. The new Jill no longer thought as this past person did, nor did she feel any obligation to her either. With the 'old Jill' went the anger and stress of that person and old hurts and in its stead, the new Jill saw life in a gentler, more understanding way. In her case, this was largely an emotional change that followed on from her physical brain change: the damage to the left side of her brain (the judgement/analytical part) meant, for the first time, that there was scope for her to think using the right side of her brain (inner peace, joy compassion). She realised she had the choice to live differently, to draw on inner peace, joy, compassion and other right brain sided responses. Then she realised — she was almost blindsided by this knowledge — that the choice to live more joyously and less judgementally had always been available to her.

She hadn't needed her stroke to bring about this positive change, but until it happened she had lived in a way that was blind to the possibilities of a more 'right sided life'. Her stroke had removed the blinkers, revealing what a right sided life could be like, after which she consciously put aside some of her past (predominantly left sided) ways of viewing life. This, in fact, was her 'stroke of insight' that formed the title of her book. This insight has valuable implications for all of us, in her words: *that peace is only a thought away, and all we have to do to access it is silence the voice of our dominating left mind.* We can walk away from past restrictions. Other ways of viewing life are available to us, if only we look.

It is an amazing insight. This clarity about the way the brain works has, she says, put her in the driver's seat in a way that she wasn't before — and most of us are not. She consciously put an end to negative mind chatter (verbal abuse she calls it) that could torpedo her recovery, and, after any moment of anger or stress, consciously waited for 90 seconds before responding, knowing this is how long it takes for the chemical flow through the brain that is responsible for those emotions to dissipate. It's a powerful idea.

She also focused more consciously on the things that brought her joy and wonder. She wrote: 'I must be willing to consistently and persistently tend the garden of my mind moment by moment, and be willing to make the decision a thousand times a day.'

Constantly choosing to prune your thoughts by encouraging the good and discouraging the bad ('tending the garden of my mind') is not as easy as it sounds. Rose, my nine-year-old granddaughter reminded me of this when she said 'Kathleen, saying something bad about yourself is the same thing as swearing. You've got to put some money in the swear jar.' I often found I needed help to stay on track, with people to rescue me when I wandered off into negativity. This led to the creation of one of my favourite recovery aids, the Hope Team.

The Hope Team

The unthankful heart discovers no mercies; but the thankful heart will find, in every hour, some heavenly blessings.
Henry Ward Beecher

None of us can remember how my 'hope team' started, but I'm very pleased it did, for the concept of having your own personal hope team is a really good one. We *think* it began as a result of my friend Kate's visits during my long stay in slow stream rehab. We'd talk of the future and my (hoped for) return to normal life and talking about this vision of the future propped my hopes up when they were flagging. I think one night I turned to her and said, 'you are the Captain of my Hope Team.' And that was it. She became 'Captain Kate.'

We invited other friends to join and suddenly I had this thing we referred to as the Hope Team. We kept it small and haven't ever really articulated exactly what a hope team is. Perhaps we feared that if we said what it was, we'd put pressure on this small loosely linked group of people. But the benefits were obvious.

At the beginning, using emails, we made a list of my hopes. This also forced me to really think about what my priorities were, what I specifically wanted to achieve — other than the obvious aim of getting well again. Getting well was too general an aim. There is power in thinking through the general to smaller, more easily targeted hopes that can be pinned down to a result.

I needed to break down 'getting well again' into separate parts, so the future could become something tangible that I could visualise.

This was my list:

1. To continue to progress in my return to health

2. To find and establish my new lovely home that will facilitate me living independently

3. That the funding will appear to write and publish my book

4. That the book will help me to reinvent my professional life

Later I added another:

5. To stay open to the hope that I will attract a wonderful partner/lover into my life.

Sitting inside my room in slow-stream rehab, I have to admit that these hopes seemed to belong to another world. I was making painfully slow progress, it seemed to me. I was far from having a new home; in fact I was struggling with the reality of selling the home I loved. I did want to write a book about what I'd been through eventually, but there was nothing to suggest this was even a remote possibility.

I can see, looking back, that I was honing my thinking about the future; how I wanted to live, what shape my new life could take. What I ended up writing down were five hopes of great importance. Having a support team linked to these hopes meant I had people to share my hopes with, who would help me to keep going and issue rebukes when I wandered off. They were like a mix between a cheer squad and a very loving umpire! We need support, all of us.

Kate recalls, 'My job in the Hope Team was to keep Kathleen's hopes up. There were times when Kathleen would lose hope, which is completely understandable; of course you're allowed to have days when it's too hard! Personally, I used to sometimes think that I didn't know what Kathleen's future would hold, but I am astounded by her extraordinary progress and what's happened. It's due to her courage and commitment to the future and the hope she is determined to maintain. She has an amazing resilience of spirit.'

The Hope Team also encouraged me to do something that many women find difficult, to put my needs and myself first, to make my hopes the priority. Kate recalls, 'It was my observation, over many years of friendship, that Kathleen often put her family before herself. Indeed, at the time of her stroke she was dedicating an enormous amount of time and energy to both her ageing parents and her lobbying about Angelman Syndrome. And I know that it distressed her that she couldn't give more to her daughters and their needs once she'd had a stroke. So I saw my role as being to remind her of the need to put herself first; she needed to free herself from a sense of obligation in order to get on with the work of recovery.'

The Hope Team relied a lot on phone calls and emails. People are busy and visiting isn't always possible, but I had access to my team whenever I needed it. So when I moved out of rehab I could share huge moments of progress, such as the night I first made soup for my daughter who had come to visit, as well as the not so good moments. It's sometimes just nice to have people to share things with. In April 2014, I emailed this to my team:

Quite a day today. As you know, I'm in residential rehab again for the next four weeks. With the help of two physios, I walked up and down a huge flight of stairs. Also had lots of walking practice. I walked to and from breakfast group and showering myself. I got a new orthotic and practised putting it on myself and succeeded. I did my washing and hung it up in my bathroom.

Then I went to see my cardiologist. I wasn't really surprised when she observed after watching me walk to the bed, that I should not be living on my own as I am not safe, as she is the doctor who commented that a further stroke would kill me so I need not worry about having one! I am tired of the negativity of medicos. That's why I need you all!

The replies included: 'I felt tired just reading what you did yesterday — hope there are some 'prouds' in there for you! Wow! .... maybe cardiologists deal with other people's hearts to make up for having none themselves! And Huge congratulations on walking up and down stairs and putting on your own orthotics and for doing and hanging out your own washing. These are massive leaps in your world. As for the comment of your cardiologist — words fail me!'

Kate: 'The tyranny of distance meant the main way I supported Kathleen to hold on to her hope was by phone. Sometimes she would ring and just say, can I talk? For her 60th birthday I had given Kathleen a set of Goddess Cards, which I see as a mixture of playful and the deeply real. So she would flag that she had a dilemma and I'd encourage her to think about what she was looking for guidance on, then I'd shuffle the cards until she told me to stop.

'The value in having this little structure was that it gave us reflection time and a safe environment, which is so important to reflection, where we went that step further in a way that was a bit spiritual and a bit playful. It was a way of giving ourselves time and space to think through with a bit of process. We're both deeply sceptical (and the cards are not for the hardened cynic!) but we've been gobsmacked by how on the mark they can be. There was only one reading we did that didn't speak to us at all.'

Over time my Hope Team developed and we changed its name to the Belief Team. By then I was living almost independently behind Petrina and Gordon's house and no longer captive in rehab, so I had progressed (to some extent) to being able to take my fate into my own hands. Some of the Hope Team's hopes had come to pass. Now I needed to believe that I could manifest even more, or, as one member of the team suggested, I had moved out of the more wistful hope stage of early recovery and into the more robust world of stronger belief. We all agreed at that stage that belief seemed more appropriate than hope.

In preparation for the change from hopes to beliefs, I came up with a list of areas in which I wanted to progress. I thought carefully about each before sending it on to my team as I knew each would need a lot of energy, and I didn't have much. I was still suffering from fatigue and couldn't afford to waste effort. But the process was timely. I was in residential rehab undergoing four weeks of intense therapy, so thinking about 'Why am I doing this?' seemed entirely appropriate.

This is what I wrote:

- Creating a new home that facilitates my independence and that is warm and welcoming for my family and friends
- Enjoying the beauty of nature daily
- Being healthy and vital so I really enjoy my life
- My professional life reinvented and reinvigorated
- My book creating a revenue stream for me and Vicki and helping other stroke survivors and their loved ones
- Spending lots of happy family time with Emma, Piet, Asher, Rose, Jack, Lucinda and Richard
- Social life flourishing including ballet, opera, concerts, golf, bridge
- Relationship, my wonderful soulmate finding me. Creating a happy and fulfilling life together.

Kate and I then worked on a final version and this is it.

The Kathleen Jordan Belief Team

Leader:	Kathleen
Team Members	Liz, Kate, Vicki and Pam
Kathleen's Vision	I am manifesting progress in all areas of my life, and in particular:

- I am creating a new home that facilitates my independence and that is warm and welcoming for my family and friends
- I am enjoying the beauty of nature daily
- I am healthy and vital so I really enjoy my life
- My professional life is reinvented and invigorated
- My book is creating a revenue stream for Vicki and me and is helping other stroke survivors and their loved ones
- I am spending lots of happy family time with Emma, Piet, Asher, Rose, Jack, Lucinda and Richard
- My social life is flourishing including ballet, opera, concerts, golf, bridge
- My wonderful soul mate is finding me and we are creating a happy and fulfilling life together

Purpose of the Belief Team	To help Kathleen keep belief in her vision and attain her goals.
Team Objectives	To support Kathleen:

1. To continue to make progress towards returning to good health. For example, to be walking with confidence around her home without supervision

2. To find and establish her lovely new home that will facilitate her living independently

3. To believe that the funding will appear for the writing and publishing of the book

4. To believe that the book will help her reinvent her professional life

5. To help her stay open to the belief that she will attract a wonderful partner/lover into her life

Operating principles That team members

1. Commit to having one-on-one time with Kathleen at least once a month (be that face-to-face or by phone) to support and encourage her with her vision and goals

2. Contact each other as we choose.

When Vicki pointed out to me that I needed to mention sex and love in this book, I emailed my freshly minted Belief Team, telling them how uncomfortable the idea made me feel and seeking their help. Their encouragement gave me the strength to overcome my feelings of vulnerability — they were a personal sounding board, a trusted panel, whose comments I always knew were made with my best interests at heart.

Celebrations and prouds

Gratitude is the most exquisite form of courtesy.
Jacques Maritain

On the second anniversary of my stroke, there was a knock on my door and a delivery of a huge bouquet of red roses. *In acknowledgement of two years of courage and progress* read the note from my sister Petrina and her wonderful family. A card and a bottle of champagne arrived from another of my sisters celebrating my 'three' years of progress. It was a mistake — she was a year ahead of herself but I understood. With everything she and my family had done for me and my parents in that time, it probably felt more like three years than two! My daughters rang to let me know again how glad they were to have their mother back, and how pleased and inspired they felt by my progress.

If you want to shoot down grief, celebration is a great way to do it. I had the choice on the first anniversary to either mark the year's losses with grief, or celebrate the fact I was still alive. Naturally, grief crept in but a life affirming celebration kept me on track. It's a choice you have to make, and the choice needs to be in favour of life. Therefore, celebrate.

We are a family of celebrators and nothing gets in our way. It brings us together and strengthens our bonds. It focuses our thoughts on the good times, when the bad times threaten to push all before them. And that is why, even on the first anniversary of my stroke, we gathered for a lovely lunch. In the face of death, had I not survived? I credit our celebrations as a huge factor in my recovery.

By the time of my third anniversary, I was in the midst of some moments of wondering if I wanted to survive. I was tired of it all. In these moments, resilience means acknowledging that these feelings will pass and using courage to get through. It's tough and takes courage. But celebration again came to my rescue. The one we had that time was so special that my moments of self-pity seemed pitiful in comparison. My daughters told me how grateful they were that I was alive, that they still had me, the mother they knew and loved. Knowing they nearly lost me is more than they can bear to think about. How could I feel ungrateful in the face of that?

Petrina's message on my card that day ended, *With deep appreciation of your courageous spirit — stronger than ever these past three years. We love having you live with us, All our love Petrina and the tribe.* These loving words from my family have inspired me to keep going, achieving more milestones. They were as good as therapy.

My daughter Lucinda was to marry Richard in February 2012, but we were then all still juggling the many dire predictions after the stroke. They postponed that celebration to November so I could be, in Lucinda's words, 'the guest of honour.' In the weeks prior to the wedding, my dear friend Diana visited from England and took on the role of my carer. For a wonderful few days we lived in a beautiful city apartment, kindly lent by my friend Margaret. Those special 'pre-wedding days' meant I didn't have to attend my daughter's marriage coming straight from the rehab unit. The apartment was an eye-opener after a year of institutionalisation and it was there that I began to feel strongly that there could be life beyond rehab.

Their wedding was the happiest of times, just as Emma's wedding had been years earlier. Later I stayed up late, soaking up the happiness as people shared dinner and dancing in a lovely restaurant. In the following days I went to see *Madame Butterfly* with Diana and visited Port Fairy with my family. If you don't celebrate these moments of friendship and celebration, what is the purpose of all the recovery struggle? This is the payoff and it gives a surge of energy to be amongst the good things of life again.

I remember with gratitude and pride the celebrations we shared when Lucinda submitted her PhD thesis, 'Seeking Place. Young people, homelessness and violence' to Monash University. I subsequently found out that her final draft had been returned by her supervisor without any corrections at all, which is, I am told, amazing. We celebrated again when she received her doctorate. In her acknowledgements, Lucinda expressed gratitude to many people, including, of course, her partner Richard. But, typical Lucinda, she acknowledged everyone who had helped, including her dog Millie Moo, surely one of the few dogs in the world to be thanked for their contribution to a doctoral thesis. 'Thanks to you Millie my constant study buddy, for keeping my feet warm during thunderstorms and reminding me of what is important in life — playing ball and going for walks in the sunshine.'

Anniversaries can be profound in many ways. Four years after the car crash, Christine Durham visited the lamp-post her car had ended up wrapped around when it was hit by another car. It was the place where everything changed for her. There were still traces of paint on the pole. Standing in the rain, she put her arms out and hugged the post. She wrote, 'From that moment on, I felt something inside me start to heal.'

Another form of celebration is what my Hope Team calls 'prouds'. A proud is, as the name suggests, a moment when you stop and take time to feel proud of something. They are good to use whenever you achieve something new. In the tsunami of difficulties that follow trauma, it's easy to focus on what you *can't* do and to let slide the tiny moments which, added together, accumulate to form progress. Kate called these moments, simply, 'prouds' and I can't think of a better word. Prouds can be tiny, but if you stop to recognise them they add to the credit side of a ledger that, at times, can feel all too full of debits. I recommend noticing any 'prouds' in any given day. They're like noticing how good our lives are, instead of focusing on the day's worries.

Prouds also clock progress. Some weeks or months, progress can seem glacial, or non-existent, but if you look at your list of prouds, progress becomes evident. I like to look back over last week or last month's prouds, and notice that what was a proud a few weeks ago has become routine the next. This is the way the small steps to progress work. I think of them as being like small children, the offspring of celebration and gratitude. They might be small but their cumulative effects are very big, if you just stop and notice each one.

As I approached my third anniversary, my prouds included staying with Lucinda and Richard for two nights (in the house I was originally going to live in) and finding that I managed very well walking around their home and coping with a new routine. When staying at Port Fairy, unlike on previous visits, the wheelchair was left parked while I walked around.

People and places of inspiration

The greatest glory in living lies not in never falling,
but in rising every time we fall.
Nelson Mandela

In 1945, holocaust survivor, Victor Frankl sat down to write his memoir. Within nine days he had completed *Man's Search for Meaning* which has now been translated into more than 20 languages and, by the time of Frankl's death in 1997, had sold over 10 million copies. His message was to show the reader 'by concrete example that life holds a potential meaning under any conditions, even the most miserable ones.'

His experience at Auschwitz showed him that 'the great task for any person is to find meaning in his or her life.' When he looked at the survivors around him, he realised that hope (or lack of hope) was as important to people's survival prospects as food and medicine (or their lack). Harold S Kushner wrote in the introduction to the 2008 edition, 'Forces beyond our control can take away everything you possess except one thing, your freedom to choose how you will respond to the situation. You cannot control what happens to you in life, but you can always control what you will feel and do about what happens to you.' I'd read Frankl's book before setting up my business and used his approach to thinking as a path for my own. Now I really needed to go back to him and people like him, and see what they did for far more crucial reasons.

Frankl was imprisoned by something that was almost entirely beyond his control — and yet in that 'almost' he found the key. He believed that his greatest freedom was his ability to choose how he responded to the situation he was in. His captors could not control his thoughts, and therein lay his survival and in time, his future. From this a new life could be built.

I had to be the same. It is a philosophy I used a lot in my leadership coaching. It wasn't always easy to keep choosing the right thoughts in the early days post stroke but it is what has given me the strength to keep on going. If he could do it, why couldn't I?

I thought a lot about people who had overcome worse than I was going through, like Frankl. Fortunately, I'd read a lot of books written by those people in my working life, so the library was already 'in my mind.' After the stroke, I didn't have the concentration or energy required to read. But I could remember what they'd written, what they'd learned about struggle. The gold nugget inside their words is that they come from experience. These aren't thoughts written to inspire people by psychologists and motivators. They are the real deal and that gives them great weight.

Frankl went on to become a professor of psychiatry and neurology, having survived four concentration camps. *When we cannot change a situation, we are challenged to change ourselves,* he wrote, which is an astonishing insight. *Transform a tragedy into a triumph, a predicament into a human achievement. Suffering ceases to be suffering when it finds meaning. Suffering is not necessary to finding meaning, but meaning is possible despite suffering.* As he says, there are many potentialities in every situation and the one that is actualised is done so by choice; we made a decision. And at the point of that decision lies our choice.

The belief that finding meaning in your life is the great task for each of us has resonance with the current positive psychology movement. I'll look at that movement later. Humans need something to live for that is genuine and authentic, not just related to money and its trappings. Meaning can come, says Frankl, from work, from love, or from courage in a difficult time. It's about being aware of *what can be done* in a given situation, so that even in suffering one can choose to be responsible.

A friend of mine, Bernadette, writes about this in a slightly different way. 'It is those moments in life [those that are dealt to us] that give us a special opportunity, an opportunity to tap into that profound part of our being which reveals to us in a unique way, a level of strength, confidence and faith we have within ourselves that we did not know of at the time.'

Frankl tells a story of being beaten and falling down in the snow and in the midst of his suffering and abuse he says to himself, 'One day I'll tell this story to a room full of people.' He held that vision and ended up telling his story to a room of 2,000 people and not the 20 he'd originally envisaged. It makes me go goose-bumpy every time I think about it.

My vision was to write a book, and I found this gave meaning to what I went through. It meant my experience could become a story that I could tell to help others, rather than just a terrible situation I was forced to endure. In that way my suffering found a meaning and I didn't surrender to the situation. It didn't mean that, given the choice, I would have chosen to have a stroke, far from it. That was simply life in action and I couldn't control that part. I could only control my reaction to it.

As life moved on, so did the meaning, keeping pace with my expanding situation. What gave me hope one year was not enough the next. I see this as progress. Frankl writes that meaning should be looked at in terms of a person's life at a given moment. It will naturally change as our lives change. So I kept looking for meaning at every stage, while retaining my vision for a book. I believe, as many people do, that holding a strong vision for the future gives energy to a situation and can attract the right people to help me achieve my aim.

Which is exactly what happened with this book. Determined as I was to write a book about my experiences, I had no idea how to go about it or where to start. Then, one night, an email arrived from a man I hadn't seen since before my stroke. We had met in Sydney during our respective business trips, as we stayed at the same hotel. We'd share a red wine and much laughter in the hotel's executive lounge. He hadn't heard from me for a while and emailed to say he hoped I was alright. When I told him about my stroke he was greatly saddened, and when I told him I was determined to write about it, he had an answer. It led immediately to Vicki Steggall, who arrived in my life. All at once I could relax. She was handling my great desire.

Not all results come so quickly and neatly but often the answer to a situation is lying just beyond reach. Someone else may have that extra reach. It's an extension of my business philosophy to always ask the person I'm speaking to, if they can't assist me, whether they know someone else who might.

Not all inspiration and strength needs to come from the great and the good. The calming effect of nature is a human being's secret ally and so frequently overlooked that we can forget its power. Perhaps because it's freely available without effort, we so often fail to notice. But we are animals living in a manufactured environment and when we step back to our natural world, something deep inside us responds. We are home and a wounded human needs the solace of home to recover.

Nature provides perspective. It is the force against which we can measure our lives and see that all is ebb and flow, that we are surrounded by beauty even when we fail to notice. So often we wait too long to welcome it into our lives, putting our business first. It is an important healer.

Meditation, or simply relaxing and letting go, is another ally but there are times when the tranquillity inside us is just not there. I found, in the environment of the rehab unit and with loss of some brain function, that I could not meditate, or even concentrate on being 'in the now.' Peacefulness eluded me, which was a departure from what I had taught! I was unable to do as I had so often suggested others do. But, in mitigation, I could say that the noisy, unsettling environment of a rehab unit was not a conducive environment. There are times when we are too agitated to meditate, or we don't have the commitment or it's not right for us.

This is where the rose garden became my ally. I would sit in my wheelchair watching the birds wheeling overhead, the roses nodding in the breeze and find myself naturally doing what I had so struggled to do inside the building. It was uninterrupted time with a reminder of beauty and life. I could feel the gentle beneficence entering every pore in my cells. Sometimes my family would visit me there, and sometimes, the golden retriever, Buddy, would join us too.

These are places to seek out. Whether it's the local park or a corner of the garden, or a window overlooking something calming. We can't expect our brains to heal when we are surrounded by agitation. Late, far too late, hospitals are realising the healing power of a garden, or even fresh air and sunlight.

Christine Durham writes of the power of watching birds in the trees outside her window at home. During her early recovery when she was scarcely able to communicate with her own family, she watched the different families bringing up their young and the change of seasons. Nature asked nothing of her. She could just be and she felt the gentle joy of watching these birds go about their lives.

On those days when pleasure is hard to find, I sit and watch the heroics of the rabbits, chasing each other and attempting feats of escapism. Then my eyes skim over the more peaceful scene of blackbirds drinking from the birdbath at my window. Sometimes the pigeons shoo them away, but they always return to enjoy ruffling their feathers in the water. Their antics and little personalities and the natural world of the garden perform a sort of alchemy, turning despair into something easier to live with. I can feel its hold on me fracturing and releasing me. It reminds me that it will pass and that my role, in the face of despair, is to have courage.

When I was in my twenties, my mother always told me that I was the most courageous person she'd ever met. These small moments, looking at the chabbits and bringing myself around from despair to hope, are those that take the most courage. How funny that so often my companions in this struggle are rabbits and chickens, but really I have much to thank them for.

We are surrounded by blessings. If you're reading this book, then you live in an advanced society where you have somewhere safe to read, enough food to eat and a society that has safety nets should you need them. That puts you ahead of the vast majority of people on this planet. Eventually, as my tension ebbed, I found I was able to pull together small strands like this from my previous training and they were highly effective.

I have always sought out inspiration from other people and places. I have a briefcase on wheels, which I call my wheelie-bin, where I keep my inspirational resources. I have a folder of quotes that I find on the internet, some DVDs that help with my vision and focus, and cards that I used to use with my clients to prompt thoughts about people like Frankl and Nelson Mandela. Now, instead of using them on my clients, I use them for myself. Many of the quotes that I have found most powerful are in this book.

I recommend reading everything you can about people who have faced similar problems, which are really problems of character and determination, even though the circumstances are different. Write down the lines that make you stop and keep a file or even a wheelie-bin of resources for growth. The input we give ourselves is as important as the food we feed ourselves. Keep scanning, as the words you need to read tend to come up when you need them, and they can make a remarkable difference to how you work your way around a problem.

Self-compassion

Sometimes it can be hard to be kind to yourself. Recently, while playing with my nine-year-old granddaughter Rose, I made some self-deprecating comment, along the lines of, 'I am not much good at this, am I?' She admonished me, quite correctly, with, 'Saying bad things about yourself is the same as swearing. Put some money in the bad language jar.' Perhaps we should all keep a container nearby to add cash to when we are unkind to ourselves!

I find that laughter is the best way to be compassionate with oneself. I overcome my frustration with slow progress by being proud of my achievements. If all else fails, I laugh at how absurd I must look as I struggle with daily tasks.

One of the most compassionate things I do for myself is my twice-daily meditation. It helps me connect with nature and other important things in life.

It is important to nurture yourself by getting rid of all negativity in your life. This can mean making decisions about who you want in your life. This is not always easy. It can be difficult to overcome feelings of loyalty and decide it is time to move on with your own wellbeing, but you need people who are on board with you in your hopes and dreams. I struggled to do this until it became clear that to me that coping with negativity erodes energy and I needed that energy to focus on my goals. As part of this, I made the decision to stop feeling guilty if I didn't want to watch or discuss ghastly national and international events. I know I'll be more effective when I am feeling well.

Some inspirational strategies

An enthusiastic heart finds opportunities everywhere.
Paulo Coehlo

These are some of the strategies that I've called on to help me from my professional life. They only take seconds, but can turn your thinking around quickly. I see them as little helpers that I can keep in my pocket for moments when I need a lift. It's a matter of trying each and seeing which works best for you.

Building a cathedral

This strategy, called chipping stone or building a cathedral, is very simple but sometimes it's all that's needed. Basically it is about reframing your thinking: a person in medieval Florence chipping away at a piece of marble could either believe he was just chipping a lump of stone or that he was indeed building a cathedral.

Like that person, I too needed to reframe my thinking. With each exercise or attempt to sit without falling over or stand without collapsing backwards, I could think I am doing my physiotherapy and this sucks! Or I could think 'I am moving towards health and vitality.' This re-frame helped me to be more positive and driven.

Reframing the language that you use is also important. When

nurses ask, 'Which is your bad leg?' I reply, 'I don't have a bad leg, I just have an unhappy one.' I don't want my brain to hear negativity about any of my body parts as it won't help healing.

On the days when this approach seemed difficult, and there were many, I would say to myself, 'Pretend you *really are* moving towards your pre-stroke way of life'. This pretence helped fool my brain and gave me energy to continue.

Creating a full cup

This is identifying what fills your emotional cup, and then drawing on that emotional energy to focus on the task at hand. For me, music, nature and fresh air fill my emotional cup. So I had beautiful music playing in my room and whenever possible took myself outside into the fresh air and nature.

Being with family and friends also fills my emotional cup. However, I needed things that I could do for myself in the long hours when I was on my own. This is easier to do now that I am home: in rehab there were days I really struggled to think about filling up emotional cups. Now I have the chabbits to watch and children skipping in to say hello and the sun streaming in my window, and these create a very full cup most days.

Pollyanna's exercise

The quickest way to feeling happy is just to think about (and list) the things that you are grateful for. I call this the Pollyanna exercise. If you are feeling like shit with an attack of the *why me's?* then do this gratitude exercise. Even one thing that you are grateful for can alter your thinking and bring energy into your day.

The voice in your head

But there are times when that Pollyanna moment seems impossible — gratitude is just too far away from where you're at. This is when the 'voice in your head' exercise can come to the rescue. It's from Ben Zander, whose leadership DVD is called *Leadership, an art of Possibility* and I used it with clients. Ben suggests that when that voice in your head tells you that you *can't* do something (or says, there isn't a single thing to feel grateful for so why bother with that Pollyanna thing?) that you speak directly back to it. He suggests using words like *thank you for your opinion, but I'm too busy to listen right now* and politely dismiss its negative message. When I'm not in such a polite mood, I have sometimes shortened the message to *Piss off. I don't need your negative thoughts.*

We all have a negative voice that undermines us at every turn and being alert to its insidious presence is powerful. That negative voice sneaks in at all sorts of moments, such as when you find yourself colluding with medicos when they tell you that you'll never achieve something. At that moment, listen to what that voice in your head says (*if the medicos have said it, it must be right),* thank it for its viewpoint and dismiss its readiness to always agree with the worst possible outcome.

Breathing love

In my professional life I had been an accredited provider of Heartmath methodology and I had taught this to my clients. It was obvious to me that stress was getting in the way of so many people's ability to form good relationships at work, to make effective decisions and was interfering with their lives in general. Heartmath techniques gave a pathway to handle this. Unfortunately, like the cobbler whose children go barefoot, I only used them intermittently before my stroke (and I wonder if I had taken greater care of myself, could I have avoided the stroke?)

But I began to practice again, when I felt I could. An exercise I found very helpful was to focus my breathing on the chest area around my heart and imagine myself generating feelings of love and appreciation, flowing from me right across the room. This in turn increased my feelings of gratitude towards life and for all the things that had gone right, rather than brooding on what had gone wrong. It gave bodily focus to my belief that there is something to appreciate in almost any given situation, and I could feel my breathing ease and gentleness flow around my body.

The Beliefs Tree

This exercise comes from my friend and colleague Kate from AnD Leadership Consulting. I use it when my focus falters and I need to think more deeply about why I'm not progressing as I'd like. I might have done the usual things, but, nothing happens. This is where thinking about the Beliefs Tree gets me back on track — it forces me to look beneath the surface to see what is really going on.

> *Picture, if you will, a large mature tree — maybe you have a favourite tree that you can bring to mind. Then take a piece of A4 paper and draw that tree. You could then use this picture as a self-coaching exercise by calling it your Beliefs Tree.*
>
> *The purpose of the Beliefs Tree model is to bring to the spoken any unconscious beliefs that could sabotage your*

chosen path. The image of the tree is used as a metaphor for one's life, just as Kathleen and I have used it for hers on and off over the years of her rehabilitation.

The leaves and branches of her Beliefs Tree represent the visible Kathleen that we recognise her by: her glossy black hair, her beautiful smile and her sparkling eyes, and her always well-groomed appearance.

The trunk of Kathleen's Beliefs Tree represents her values. These are less visible than her physical characteristics but quickly discovered as we get to know her. And given you are reading Kathleen's book, you will know what a strongly values-driven woman she is.

What is not visible but in fact nourishes and sustains Kathleen's Beliefs Tree is the root system beneath the ground. In the metaphor, these are Kathleen's beliefs, gathered since the moment someone said, 'It's a girl' when she was born. Because she has done so much self-development over the years, many of Kathleen's beliefs are conscious and positively inform the decisions she makes. But for her, just as for all of us, some of our beliefs remain unconscious and can nonetheless be either a positive or a negative influence on the progress we make with our life choices.

As you will know from this book, Kathleen's vision for her future has been a driving force of her rehabilitation. At times when she has been dogged with doubts, she has asked if we could spend time on her Beliefs Tree so that she could identify any negative beliefs that might be getting in the way of her ongoing progress such as 'You are not strong enough,' 'You can't do this,' or 'You are not loveable.'

As you have read before in this book, quite early in her rehabilitation Kathleen began calling me the 'Captain of her

Hope Team.' This then evolved to the establishment of her Beliefs Team — a small group whose role it is to help her hold her belief in achieving her vision for her recovery. She and I worked on this vision and the set of core beliefs to support these so that when she is having a bad day or something unexpected arises that is a barrier to her progress, she can consciously return to her positive beliefs, which are listed in the Hope Team section.

Kate

Walking the labyrinth

Eighteen months after coming home, I walked a labyrinth. Prior to my stroke, I had walked the labyrinths at Grace Cathedral in San Francisco — one inside, one outside. I'd also regularly walked a labyrinth at a retreat in Arizona, where I had worked on global leadership development programs. I'd walked the Crystal Castle labyrinth each time I'd stayed with my dear friend Kate in the hills outside Byron Bay.

Like many others, I'd found the experience of walking a labyrinth to be very moving, a time of peace and reflection as I thought about life's twists and turns, joys and sorrows.

At the Grace Cathedral I had bought a wooden replica of the labyrinth (which is modelled on the famous one at Chartres Cathedral) and many times over the years since my stroke I would trace it with my finger, reliving the experience.

But I had not walked a labyrinth since my stroke. Until, that is, Petrina, Gordon and their children took me to the Community Church of St Mark, where the pastor laid a large canvas with a labyrinth drawn on it on the floor of the church. All the pews were pushed back, so the group could do a contemplative walk. I felt, well, daunted by it. Someone suggested that while others were walking it, I could colour in photocopies as the children were doing. Naturally my response was 'Bugger that! I AM going to walk it.'

Everyone else was walking the canvas barefoot, but I was allowed to keep my shoes on, as shoes and calliper were part of my necessary walking equipment. I took a deep breath and slowly and firmly started the walk. At first I wasn't convinced I'd make it. However, with each step, I felt stronger.

When you walk a labyrinth, you meditate on something important to you. Naturally, to me that was my darling Lucinda's recovery and my own improvement, so as I walked, I focused on creating a loving, healing future for both of us.

I was very concerned that I might be slowing people down. I need not have been. The man who was walking behind me told me afterwards that he found it very moving to walk behind me: 'I found your focused, purposeful steps both hypnotic and inspirational... you aided my meditative journey.'

Life felt wonderful, full of possibility. If you don't know about labyrinths I suggest you start reading about them. They are often confused with mazes, but they are quite different. With a labyrinth, the path is clearly defined right in front of you and they are designed so that you walk from the outside to the centre, slowly, along that path. The Labyrinth Society (labyrinthsociety.org) describes them as 'a single path or universal tool for personal, psychological and spiritual transformation, thought to enhance right brain activity.' They are extraordinarily peaceful and have been used as an aid to human contemplation for many centuries.

Insight writing

This is one of the most powerful ways of dealing with grief and trauma. Writing is not a natural activity for most people and there is a tendency to worry about what the end result will be like. But this is a different sort of writing, designed to free you from any inhibition or reluctance.

I suggest you simply put your pen to the paper — and start. Make sure the pen doesn't leave the paper. The first few sentences or pages might be just random words strung together, making no sense, but eventually your brain connects to the pen and words tumble out. I call it insight writing because when you free yourself from expectations, but keep that pen moving, insights occur. The best way to 'catch' them is to read your scrawl back afterwards and look for words that reappear or moments of insight that you've produced — those Aha! moments. Read them and use them to meditate on. Perhaps start with them on your next day of insight writing.

After Lucinda died, I used insight writing to help me stay sane. I just began the moment with my memories of her and let the rest flow.

Bobath therapy

Bobath is a therapy that assesses people according to their individual issues, using a problem solving approach for each patient. It doesn't assume that all people moved the same way before their stroke, or present with the same issues after.

My main issue was my perception of where I was in space. Part of this may have been because of sensory loss to the left side of my body, so that only half of my body was giving feedback to my sensory system to work out where my body was and how it was aligned. Usually the brain relies on information from many sensory receptors and each movement updates the brain about the existence of that receptor.

So, when you don't use a part of your body, the brain stops representing that part as much. This creates an issue when you then want to move that part, because when you try to send the signal to move, your brain doesn't know where the part is.

I had been immobile for such a long time (not moving my limbs around as one normally would) that my brain had difficulty knowing where my body parts were and, therefore, where the middle of my body was. As a result I always felt like I was falling and couldn't work out how to keep my balance. For people who haven't experienced this feeling, it is sometimes difficult to recognise how absolutely frightening it is to be trying to stand and walk, or even bend forward. In fact most of us are so frightened of falling forward on our faces that we usually lean back.

So the first thing that my therapist did was to make it possible for me to move parts of my body selectively, so that they could send information to the central nervous system that they existed as separate parts of the body, not just one big clump of body. As an example of 'clumping', when I tried to lift up my left arm, I would start by bending my body towards the right, whilst elevating my left shoulder to try to lift the arm, which then turned in towards the body. This body bending was my attempt to stabilise myself against the movement of the arm, but it wasn't useful because it meant that I always had to move my body to move my arm.

What I needed to learn was to keep my body up against gravity and hold it there. Once stable, it became a reference point so when I moved my arm, I could move my arm against its stability. Then I needed to learn to initiate the movement from my hand. This effectively shortened the lever from a physics point of view, making the arm lighter to lift. This required several steps. First I needed to activate my trunk and stabilise it against the perturbation caused by the weight of the arm moving. Then I needed to know where my hand, elbow, shoulder were (including my shoulder blade which helps stabilise the arm to the trunk) as separate entities, because they all move at slightly different times to create a coordinated pattern for reaching. My therapist assisted the movements, guiding them to control initiation, timing and pattern, but I actually had to perform the activity. Skilled handling is required by the therapist to stimulate the appropriate sensory receptors, which then create a demand on my nervous system to perform the movement. The advantage of their facilitation was that I didn't need to think about all of the aspects of the movement (which was far too complex in many cases), but rather feel my way through it.

Once I learnt the movement pattern, I took more and more control of all of the aspects of the movement. The goal was for me to take over the whole movement.

My therapists created a safe environment for me to stand up and explore moving through space, using objects like the backs of chairs to block me in. They also showed me where upright was, so I started to use vision just as I had pre-stroke, as a receptor to understand critical information like where vertical was. After a stroke our sensory receptors around our muscles, joints and skin, as well as our inner ear, which let us know how the line of gravity is falling, are undamaged. However, the areas that process their information may have been.

Stimulating these receptors to send as much information as

possible to the processing areas of the central nervous system puts a demand on it to find a way to work. Sometimes that stimulation needs to be very graded and slow so that you can take it in.

Once I was upright, my therapist would make me move my body through space to create this stimulation. Selective movement that helps the central nervous system identify each part of the body (not a clump) is the best way to do this. This was often quite daunting despite her standing close by, but the more I did, the better it felt. I continue to use Bobath therapy and I am grateful to Kim for her expertise.

Who am I? Passion mapping

Your success depends mainly upon what you think of yourself and whether you believe in yourself.
William J. H. Boetcker

As I have said many times — because it's a fundamental legacy of trauma — the stroke challenged my sense of identity. I had a clear belief about what my trajectory in life was likely to be, and this was a major disruption. While I know I am (mostly) the same person inside, my physical being has undeniably changed and, of course, two years in hospital and rehab cannot help but alter you. I was me, but a different me.

But in what ways was I different? Had some parts simply left the room and others stayed? Or was it a matter of degree, like an accelerated course in advanced growing up? Perhaps, shorn of unnecessary trimmings, I'd become *more* me. Or perhaps nothing really had changed other than my perception of myself — that seeing myself sitting in a wheelchair made me think about myself differently.

This was where I found a system called passion mapping to be useful. Passion mapping has been a popular tool with consultants, and one that I regularly used to help people get to the essence of who they are. At the end of the result of passion mapping sessions (which can be intense sessions of several hours each) each person produces a map containing all the most important passions in their life. The passion map you produce is called the 'signature of the soul.' Sounds simple, but for many it is a time of great revelation.

If you know what your passions truly are (surprisingly few of us do) then you know what truly inspires you, and what direction you could take your life to increase joy in life. In the passion mapping process, a trained person asks you a series of questions, forcing you to think very deeply about yourself and distil those elements that make you who you are. What makes your life worth living? What matters above all else to you? These are the realms of the passion map, and the answers are often quite different to those people had previously believed about themselves.

For many of us, there is a yawning gap between who we are and how we make our living. In personal and business terms, this has a cost, but we can't always live our passions in a way that brings in income. When I was consulting, I could see that my clients were often unclear about core issues to do with their identity. They lacked a formal yardstick they could use when asking themselves, 'How am I living? Am I living my passions?' If we have a clear idea of who we are, it enables us to bring our whole self to the workplace and use this to benefit our work and relationships.

To someone who has suffered trauma, it can be a reminder of who they are and what really matters. A passion map provides that framework, giving shape to the questions of core identity that clients could use to examine how they live in relation to their passions and, in the workplace, how they relate to others.

I trained in passion map techniques in Sydney with Peter Wallman, the inventor/founder and CEO of Passion Maps, who took me through a wonderful process to help me articulate my life aspiration statement, essentially my meaning and purpose in life statement. Then I visited New Mexico three years before my stroke and Arizona three times in the following three years. My New Mexico visit was as a passion map facilitator, working with a major global consultancy group on their leadership program. We did maps for the directors and their wives and also for them together, 'relationship maps.' It was a very privileged and sacred space to work in.

This wonderful experience also included a hot air balloon ride at dawn over and into the Rio Grande Gorge, and was followed up by four programmes in Arizona over a three-year period. In all, I facilitated about 40 passion maps in Australia (Melbourne, Canberra and Sydney) and the USA.

The best way to describe what a passion map looks like is to describe mine. It consists of a series of short phrases, called passion elements, laid out across the page to form — in my map — the shape of an exclamation mark. Everyone's shape will be different — you get to choose how you lay it out. Usually, each map contains between 15 and 24 passion elements and getting the right words for each element is critical. Among my passion elements are universal happiness, joyful intimacy and love, generosity of spirit, chance encounters, natural beauty, authenticity, grace, hope and courage, fun and laughter, a nurturing and welcoming home, dynamic vitality, leading with the heart and smelling the roses.

The next step is an envisioning process, to help you to find your life inspiration by exploring how you're going to live your passions in all aspects of your life. My life statement, which appears on my map, is 'Bringing love, generosity and inspiration to the world.' One person I knew came up with his life inspiration 'to heal the world.' His first act, afterwards, was to ring the Lebanese prime minister and offer to take in a team of consultants to strategise about how Lebanon, in tatters after war, could be reconstructed. A friend of mine found the courage to leave her job for a more high-powered one in Bahrain. Through passion mapping, they had found their meaning and purpose.

It can take a long time to unearth and articulate a person's passion elements. For example, when I did my map, I answered one of Peter's questions by saying that I loved opera and ballet. He kept questioning me. Eventually I threw my arms in the air and said 'I just love it when my emotions are soaring.' There it was, the passion element, 'emotions soaring'; a large part of the process is getting the words right. Similarly, when I named my little grandson as being of importance to me, I went on to describe a feeling of warmth and love that rose up inside me every time I thought of him. In my passion map this became 'the essence of love.'

As I said, my passion map defined my true meaning and purpose in life as *bringing love, inspiration and generosity to the world.* Naturally, when I finally made it home, I looked at my passion map to reconnect with who I was and see if I sensed any changes.

I decided to hang it on the kitchen wall of my little unit, where it hangs still. I remind myself of my meaning and purpose statement when I become upset by the thoughtless actions of some of the carers who come to look after me. I remind myself that I can bring my generosity of spirit to the situation to improve the relationship between us. I might do it grimly, but nevertheless I do it!

When I first saw my passion map after my stroke, I felt profound sadness. It accentuated a world that was no longer available to me, such as the travel that would have occurred in those years. But part of the recovery process is to see this not as a relic of the past but as an enduring statement of who you are and what you will bring to the world when you return to it again. The passion elements it contains are also what you'll use to get back again.

The map remains an important part of reminding me of who I am. I look at it and it helps me to think, 'That's me, it's still me and that's what I want to be again.' It reminds me of what I wish to be more of. When my identity feels slippery, it's there. It has helped me remember and salute who I am. Some of the processes I taught as a consultant in the years before my stroke have fallen away in importance to me, while others have shown that they have true value. I would put passion mapping into the second category.

Even in my sad rehab room, people would always say it felt so warm and welcoming — my passion element of 'nurturing and welcoming home' on display. My belief is that life is full of encounters that can change everything — if you let them. A belief which has led to so many wonderful things, including getting this book written, appears as 'infinite possibility and chance encounters' on my passion map. The kookaburra, whose joyful supremacy in nature I so love, became my passion element for love of the natural world.

After the stroke, a counsellor asked me if there was anything I felt I should add to my map. I realised that I needed hope and courage more than I used to. I had had both, but they now belonged on my map, where they are now.

Here are some passion questions to help start the process of thinking through your passions:

Think of a time when you were at your most passionate.

1. What were you doing?
2. How did it make you feel?
3. How would others have described you?
4. How connected did you feel to others at the time? Would they have known this?
5. Did you thank them for being part of this experience?
6. Did you feel optimistic?
7. Did you feel at peace with the world?
8. With your life choices?

What are my strengths?

The quality of our expectations determines
the quality of our actions.
Andre Godin

Another technique I used to help clients develop healthy relationships and make effective decisions was to help them reflect on their strengths and use them in their lives. I believe I am blessed to have been able to take over 300 people through such a process.

Our passions and our strengths are sources of natural, well-spring energy. If we work with them, we can ease the path ahead of us.

The notion of working with our personal strengths derives from the positive psychology movement (not to be confused with positive thinking). Martin Seligman, known as the father of the positive psychology movement, believes that we should focus on making healthy choices for our lives based on our strengths, using what we already have in order to make the most of our lives, to 'flourish.' With colleagues, Seligman identified the 24 most common human strengths, which can be grouped under the six broad virtues of wisdom, courage, humanity, justice, temperance and transcendence.

These human strengths include (and you probably won't be surprised to read them) curiosity, open-mindedness, love of learning, hope, appreciation of beauty, gratitude, humour, self-regulation, fairness, leadership, forgiveness and mercy, humility and modesty, kindness, love, bravery and persistence. We know, and have known for centuries, that these character strengths are part of the human make-up that tends to lead to a 'life well led.' We don't have all of them in equal supply, in fact we are likely to have four or five that we are naturally stronger in than others and yet we may not easily be able to articulate which these are. Seligman has devised a questionnaire (www.authentichappiness.org) process to help people identify what their personal keys or 'signature strengths' are. He also wrote about how we can use these to make healthy choices.

Let me explain. Before my stroke, my signature strengths were:

- *Ability to love and be loved*
- *Courage and perseverance*
- *Appreciation of beauty and excellence*
- *Gratitude and generosity of spirit*
- *Curiosity and interest in the world*

Let's look at 'gratitude'. Seligman defines this: 'You are aware of the good things that happen to you, and you never take them for granted. Your friends and family members know that you are a grateful person, because you always take the time to express your thanks.' Henry Ward Beecher, in a quote I really like, puts it slightly differently: 'The unthankful heart discovers no mercies; but the thankful heart will find, in every hour, some heavenly blessings.'

When I looked at my situation, the things I was grateful for seemed obvious. I was so grateful that my daughters came to be with me as soon as they could get there. And grateful that I was at the Royal Children's Hospital when it happened and that Dr Terry Dwyer's quick thinking got me to the Royal Melbourne Hospital's emergency ward very quickly.

I am also grateful for the expertise of my surgeon, Dr Michael Wong. He operated on my brain and saved my life. He also was very kind, keeping Emma and Lucinda informed of my progress. It is beyond my understanding that many months later he was so brutally stabbed in the forecourt of a hospital on his way to work. I am grateful that he is alive and is now back at work, so others can benefit from his expertise as I did. I am also overwhelmingly grateful for the fact that I'm still the same person, that the essence of Kathleen is the same post-stroke. My daughters still have their mother, with the same values, with the same importance given to family and friends.

So it seemed to me there was much to be grateful for. But how could I use gratitude to support my recovery?

Actually, gratitude helped me through some tough times. If a nurse was less than kind, I reminded myself that I was fortunate to have the care I needed for my recovery, and instantly felt calmer by focusing on the big picture, rather than the petty moment. In the times I felt like giving up the struggle, I would remember all the family and friends who had supported me thus far. My gratitude for them and their efforts kept me going. Gratitude kept me focused on the good and calmed my heart.

Another of my key strengths is called 'Courage and Perseverance.' I draw on that every minute of every day just to keep going and to continue to defy the dire predictions of the medicos. I have applied my courage and perseverance to making a full recovery. A friend of mine, Bernadette, when learning about my situation, wrote: 'I knew that if anyone had the strength and tenacity to look this straight in the eye and challenge it with all her might, then that would be her.' The courage she was describing was one of my signature strengths, but any of the 24 common strengths brings its own particular support to the situation, so long as we are aware of which ones we have and decide to use them.

Knowing what our key strengths are allows us to cut straight to the core of what we have available in our personal 'tool box'. We struggle less because we are using our strengths, not trying to make progress using a quality we actually don't have much of. It also reminds us of who we are, and that we *are* strong in certain ways. We can then ride that strength each day and use it to think ourselves out of difficult situations. It may even be that if you change directions in your life after stroke, you use your key strengths to shape that future. Perhaps creativity has lain hidden behind another career and now can find its way out.

I know that humility is *not* one of my key strengths. I have always found it troublesome and once I had a business of my own, I had to drop it to the bottom of my strengths list. Going into an organisation and being humble didn't help me succeed — I had to project confidence. After the stroke, I also wondered if humility wouldn't see me colluding with the medicos who said I wouldn't get better. I need something stronger, like a full-on rush of determination, backed up by the 'ability to love and be loved' to give me strength. There was no point in me bringing my wobbly strengths to the fore in my recovery because they would not have been strong enough to be my ally.

In the end, everyone who lives a good life, which does include suffering, analyses their life, and knows they must choose meaning in life. Maintaining a 'Why me?' attitude beyond a certain point is to ask a question which has no answer and, more importantly, close the door to more beneficial thinking about your situation. We all have a different mix of character strengths, but they contribute to our making wise choices and using our will wisely. The result is a good and wise life, a life where we set the direction and are not emotionally knocked from pillar to post by events. It will also, according to research, be a longer life, perhaps because it works so well for us.

Another benefit is that it connects us with the world. We are social animals, undoubtedly the most social on the planet, moving amongst strangers every single day. When we take the focus off ourselves and connect to the world, we find many reasons to hope, share and take comfort and much more. We are freed of our own situation and allow others to help us and to see ways we can help them, restoring our dignity, sense of worth and human connectedness.

To stay connected, we need a robust sense of self. Understanding what our key strengths are builds that sense of self. The obvious person we think about in this sense is Nelson Mandela, who lived by his strengths, creating a well-lived life from the most desperate situation.

An exercise using passions and strengths

- Ask your loved one two questions. Firstly, ask them for examples of when in the past they have seen you at your most passionate. Prompt them with your own ideas. It might have been when you were playing with your grandchildren, having friends over for dinner, watching your favourite sport etc. Make a list of these passions.

- Secondly, ask them what they think your key strengths are, using the list provided in the appendix. Make a list of these.

You might find this exercise confronting, as it will bring into sharp focus what you have lost for the moment. However, your loved ones will be encouraged by the fact that you are thinking positively about who you are and who you want to be again.

The next part of the exercise we will call 'Who I am?'

- Ask someone close to you to help you go through all the strengths and passions that your loved ones have identified. Discuss these and come up with your own list of five key passions and five key strengths. Then ask those close to you if this reminds them of you before the event that changed your life.

Let's call this list 'Attributes that sum up your essence.'

Now the fun part starts.

- Each day select an attribute and decide to 'act as if' the whole day. What I mean is if you have identified 'a sense of humour' as that day's key attribute, then all day decide to laugh at all the difficulties you encounter. This could be meals arriving with lids on that you can't remove, other patients interfering with your peace and quiet or the frustrations of trying to be mobile in a world that doesn't cater for you.

- Do this for a week then ask your loved ones if they see any difference in your mood or your demeanour. Importantly, take the time to reflect how you are feeling about the future now. Has it changed the way you think?

The more you focus on different attributes, the more you will see that a future is possible. As I write, I am vacillating between hope and despair. I recognise how far I have come with my rehabilitation, but I know how much further I have to go. So I draw on one of my key attributes — courage — and I act *as if* I can do it just by having the determination to do it.

Goal setting

Wouldn't it be wonderful?
To walk to the side gate without a wheelchair?

My goal setting has taken many forms. In the early days, in the stroke ward, my goals tended to be set by my ever-vigilant family, as I wasn't able to think clearly. They were extremely basic, related to physical recovery and included survival itself, dual continence, communicating, swallowing, coping with left side neglect and sitting up without falling over.

In this period of goal setting, I was fortunate to have family members who were very supportive. One of my sisters, the trained nurse, kept the nurses looking after me on their toes with regard to toileting and continence, while another helped communication with a pen, paper and a word board and also started me on strategies for my left side neglect.

And yet, my friend Liz assures me that it was in the stroke ward that writing a book first became a project. I look back and the little I can remember is dark indeed. Maybe psychosis was a safe place to be. When reality cleared around me, my response was, 'What the hell?' I call it my 'What the hell period.' Some stages you just can't jump.

I was oblivious to the severity of my situation and probably a bit blasé about my recovery prospects. I'd had a hysterectomy 20 years before and had bounced back very quickly. I had had a hip replacement 10 years earlier and again had come through quite quickly. Although I was frightened when I had the stroke, I saw it as a nuisance that I would soon overcome.

Hence my own goal setting was somewhat unrealistic. I expected too much. But as the medicos colluded in this thinking, agreeing that I was indeed being unrealistic, so my determination grew that I would 'show the buggers!'

The rehab wards were where I started to set my own goals, in consultation with occupational therapists and physiotherapists. I was absolutely determined to get my old life back, and the only way to do it was by tiny increments. I set goals like being able to sit without falling over, then some time later to be able to drive my electric wheelchair safely, including not bumping into walls.

Smaller goals led to bigger results. Working with the physiotherapists, my small goals included being able to stand supported without fainting, then to take steps between the rails. Initially, I had to wear a hoist but felt so happy when I could actually take a few steps. Then I wanted to walk with the aid of a four point stick. This meant I had to improve my balance so did lots of standing exercises where I would place objects on different levels of shelves.

I was also working with a speech therapist. My goal was to get the left side of my face, which had dropped with the stroke, back to normal. This required lots of exercises, including awareness that I had to stop dribbling on the left side of my mouth and not to let food build up in my left cheek. Visualising the unattractive image of myself dribbling and dropping food was a good spur!

At two years, my goal was to feel stronger and overcome the fatigue I struggled with. I also wanted to have the confidence to walk without someone nearby, as recent falls had rocked my self-confidence. I was drawing — as so often was the case — on my key strength of courage. It was frightening to stand and to try to walk. When I was home, I fell several times and needed to alert people with my mCareWatch to help me up again. Each time I fell, I lost confidence but having goals and drawing on courage helped overcome that.

Once home, my goal was to prepare food for my daughters, like I had so many times in the past. It made the simple bowl of soup I produced a profound experience. I was back to being a person who could entertain and feed people.

Now I want to walk confidently around my unit and get out of a car on a curb — not needing a flat surface, and to walk to taxis without needing my wheelchair. It sounds small, but we all marvel that I can entertain such thoughts, coming from where I did.

On the 'higher' level, I had a goal to make a difference to others. I thought writing a book would be the way to do this but soon realised that making a difference was setting myself an onerous task. I thought about it more, really focusing, and realised that what was important to me was 'making a contribution.' This felt lighter than 'making a difference' and I could see that my book was indeed a contribution. We all need to have a sense of contributing to something larger than ourselves and reminding myself of that has helped me to focus in other ways too. If a goal simply seems too far off or too impossible, analyse it to see what you really meant when you set that goal. There's nothing wrong with trimming it to something you can achieve.

Happiness and kindness

In the weeks after my stroke, happiness seemed a forlorn hope. Would I ever be happy again? How do we rebuild happiness when we have been exiled from the world we spent our lives building?

There are methods than can help, and as a leadership coach I had better access to these than many. The latest thinking on happiness is that it isn't a feeling of being ecstatic (I think anyone over a certain age realises this, as nice as feeling ecstatic is!) but rather the sense of wellbeing that comes from having key aspects of our life and thinking in place. In Martin Seligman's book, *Authentic Happiness,* and on his website, www.authentichappiness.sas.upenn.edu, there is much discussion of a concept called PERMA. This stands for:

Positive Emotions

Engagement

Positive **R**elationships

Meaning and Purpose

Accomplishment

Achieving a state of PERMA is available to all of us. For instance, positive emotions can be fed by experiencing gratitude. Unsurprisingly, it all comes from inside. I recommend the book and the site.

Kindness

How strange that I should have to include a section on

kindness, as if it isn't obvious how important it is. When I look back over these years and ask myself what really stood out, it was acts of kindness. Whether it was the kitchen staff in rehab who did so many caring things for me after my parents died, or a stranger who smiled, or a taxi driver who cared enough to make my journey comfortable and welcoming, the cumulative effect of all these acts was powerful in my recovery.

We all know that an act of kindness spreads and endures, giving courage and strength in our normal life. As stroke closes your world around you, so everything within it is amplified. The words or actions of others loom large and even small tokens of kindness can act as a life rescue.

Just as my earliest — and most abiding — memory of the stroke was of the kindness of the people around and of the ambulance people, so Jill Bolte Taylor recalls the kindness of the medic in the ambulance. His compassion and touch, his gentleness, she called priceless. I felt the same about the lovely nurse in slow stream rehab who said to me, 'Kathleen, you're going to be fine. You're going to walk out of here and I'll be the one crying and cheering you on.' I thought of her words over and over. I told people about it for many months and still now I see her face and hear her words.

There was an amazing nurse on my stroke ward who treated me with such kindness and respect that I'm sure I'll never forget her. Lucinda was concerned that my hair hadn't been washed in a long time and this nurse made sure it was washed. The same nurse came and sat down beside Lucinda one night outside the ward and gave Lucinda her chocolate bar. 'Here', she said, 'you look like you need this.' Her kindness changed the night for Lucinda, knowing that someone like this was caring for her mother.

Other small but important acts of kindness eased my way. Trischa, my accountant, took over all my financial affairs and insisted on continuing even when I came home, which eased the burden on Lucinda and me. Kate and Rob, who had helped me to create a tranquil Japanese garden at my home, kept the garden looking lovely so I could relax knowing it was being tended with love and care. My niece Lydia and her partner Tim lived in the house and I could relax knowing that it was being cared for. And my long term remedial masseuse, Gael, visited me in rehab and after, imparting the bliss of her expert massages.

Christine Durham wrote about the courage needed to tackle the life she lived after her car accident, having to accept the repetition of difficulty and the knowledge that this would be her life. Encouragement, the giving of courage, was critical, she wrote, 'a smile, kindness, empathy, these things were so important and gave encouragement.' As she knew, kindness supports us when we are fragile with loss; loss of identity, loss of confidence and sometimes loss of hope.

Love and intimacy

Being deeply loved by someone gives you strength.
While loving someone deeply gives you courage.
Lao Tzu

I married a man very much older than myself. We married in England and later came to live in Australia with our two daughters. As a very traditional Englishman, he found it a difficult transition. It didn't work out as we'd hoped and we divorced. He returned to England, sadly dying when our daughters were in their early twenties. They were much too young to lose their father and were with him when he died, bravely sorting out his affairs.

As we saw in the chapter on strengths, the capacity to love and be loved is one of my top five signature strengths, according to the survey of character strengths used in positive psychology. In that survey, the capacity to love and be loved is described as, 'You value close relations with others, in particular those in which caring and sharing are reciprocated. The people to whom you feel most close are the same people who feel most close to you.'

It is very apparent throughout this book that I am blessed with a great deal of love in my life. It will also be apparent that at present I do not have an intimate partner. In spite of the sterile world of clinics that stroke patients spend much of their life in, and the loss of privacy that we have to endure, we are still sexual beings. While being known for my independence, being in a relationship has always been an important part of my sense of self — in particular, having someone to give to, emotionally, physically and spiritually. This lack of a special someone since my stroke has at times left me with a huge ache in my whole being. I need to feel loved, wanted and cherished. This is something I was very clear about before my stroke. Increasingly now there are times I yearn for a strong pair of arms around me, someone to tell me 'You are doing well, you are triumphing over a shit situation and I love you.'

I felt this most acutely when my parents died. I was alone and in a rehab unit. I longed to snuggle down in bed with a wonderful lover, to be held close. This is a feeling I've frequently had in the years since my stroke. A fulfilling sex life has always been important to me and I miss it. Whilst I have a great deal of love and happiness in my life, I long to share a special intimacy with a loving partner, just like anyone else, and to give and receive love for mutual pleasure and happiness.

Who doesn't? Romantic love is the great soother of life, the subject of more literature and poetry than any other subject. It is both necessary for the survival of the species and for our emotional happiness. As lovers, we snuggle, kiss and touch, just like a mother does to her baby. We are wired for touch and intimacy, unless we were unfortunate not to have experienced it as a baby.

I wonder, if I had had a life partner at the time of my stroke, how much less my anxiety might have been, how much more laughter and confidence would have been shared along the way? I would have returned home to someone who loved me, without the hideous threat of a nursing home hanging over me all the time. My family were beyond wonderful, but they rightly have their own lives. Some things cannot be fulfilled anywhere other than within that life partnership, that wonderful sharing of aid, comfort and acceptance. The things you know about each other that no-one else does. The love that continues beyond illness and calamity.

The other great benefit of a loving partner is their ability to push you on. One of my sisters, whose work brings her into contact with people after stroke, has noticed that the most miraculous post stroke recoveries usually occur with those fortunate enough to live with someone who will say, *no, you do it!* They also benefit from the confidence that another presence gives and I know that when I fall (which I do in the manner of a huge, dead weight) I lack confidence for a time afterwards. The presence of another person would ease that fear.

It's a two-way street. Family don't want to always be the ones to push and I need to be able to spread any requests for help. A partner bridges those situations. They also notice the changes, which can be hard to do yourself!

I can't help but fear that my chances of finding love have been diminished by the stroke. Not only am I out in life less, but I worry that I have less to offer. Images from the past of playing golf together or going for long walks along the beach are now longer-term dreams — by no means impossible, but sometimes feeling a long way off. Will he be expected to do things for me above and beyond the norm? Would *I* choose me? These are thoughts I scarcely dare articulate. However I firmly believe there is a wonderful person out there for me. Eventually, I will be the partner I long to be and we will play golf together, go for walks along the beach. We will travel, love, laugh and share life's joys and sorrows. It is part of my plan to find a partner and to be a partner.

Challenge yourself

Start by doing what's necessary; then do what's possible; and suddenly you are doing the impossible.
St Francis of Assisi

One of the after-effects of stroke can be confusion relating to memory. Just as happens in Alzheimer's (alarmingly), I found I could forget where I had put something down a few minutes ago, but remember songs I had not heard since being a school student and sing along, word perfect.

But it's not Alzheimer's and what I needed to do was to get my brain functioning again. I longed to return to playing bridge. Before my stroke, when I had been learning bridge, the person who taught me used to say that bridge would ward off dementia. As the memory loss I was suffering from seemed to have alarming similarities to dementia, I returned to bridge as quickly as I could. I knew it would exercise that part of my brain that allowed me to hold multiple and complex thoughts in my mind, and that card counting and remembering sequences would re-awaken my memory. It was also a return to the social aspects of the game.

I was blessed to have friends, Rosie and Dick, who were happy to come to visit me in slow stream rehab, bringing with them a delicious lunch and a fourth person. Their kindness made me feel I was still part of the human race and with the return of bridge came the glimmer of hope that normal life would not be too far off. (Rosie also took me on my first 'maxi taxi' ride, which was to the hairdresser, and continued to accompany me until I was able to go independently.)

In time we started playing at their home again, but it was not all smooth sailing. Some days I would feel that life really was beginning again. Other days I would struggle through a lack-lustre game, befuddled by the effect of acute fatigue, that most frustrating of side-effects of stroke.

Now I have a program on my PC called Jack to help me improve my game. I play every day in the belief that it improves my game and, more importantly my brain function. I have also joined up with memory games online, doing games and puzzles that will assist my brain to make new pathways. I enjoy playing chess with my nine-year-old nephew and eleven-year-old grandson. Needless to say, they win. However, I'm in the game!

Sudoku is wonderful for this and it helps me with my left side neglect as it forces me to seek out the left side to successfully complete each game. But it might also be tapestry, puzzles, painting, reading and singing — anything that gets your brain going and challenges that part of yourself which seems to have gone missing in action. The internet is teeming with games and puzzles that assist brain function. We are surrounded by opportunities to gain mental acuity, even from our own home.

Back in December 1996, when Jill Bolte Taylor had her stroke, the internet was in its infancy. She was helped by her amazing mother, who set about creating her own programme of mental rehabilitation for her daughter, using children's puzzles and games to constantly challenge her neurons. Jill started with simple 12 piece puzzles, but in time returned to her great creative love, making stained glass windows. This requires meticulous dexterity and awareness, but children's puzzles had been an important step, provoking her brain to recognise colour, shape, upside down from right side up, fitting them together and then using her fingers to pick up the pieces and put them in the right place.

When she realised that her medication was making her too drowsy to really accept challenges, she made the decision, where possible, to take it at night. It was a matter of looking at each problem separately, making sure that none got in the way of progress. I like the saying that 'it's not trespassing to go beyond your own boundaries.' In the post-trauma world, boundaries are there to be overcome and the more you push, the further you'll get.

Rehab for mental recovery is as critical as rehab for physical recovery. It is one thing we can take into our own hands and work on every hour of the day if we want to. Some days it will feel like waking a sleeping giant, who doesn't want to move. Others there is the delight of knowing you've made that giant twitch and that every twitch is a step forwards.

Post-traumatic growth

The strongest principle of growth lies in human choice.
George Eliot

Everything I've talked about in this part of the book has dovetailed precisely with the new psychological understanding of the effects of trauma — that it can be a pathway to growth, not just suffering. Post-traumatic growth is a new but rapidly growing area of psychological research, known sometimes as 'growth through adversity, adversarial growth, post-traumatic growth or stress-related growth.' It is based on the undeniable truth that positive development and behavioural growth can result from adverse events. Numerous stories of people gaining insight after trauma that they may never otherwise have gained are testament to this. This has been studied and found to be not merely anecdotal, but supported by research. After living through a hard time, respondents in surveys are found to be 'back to base' around three months later and, one year later, they claim to be physically and psychologically stronger.

Textbooks say its logical starting point is Frankl's observation that when we cannot change our life, we are challenged to change ourselves. And yet I think it's gentler than that, less a challenge than an awakening, an (un-asked for) chance to do what we probably should have done years earlier.

Penn State University's Growth Initiative (part of the

Positive Psychology movement) is examining how people may develop after traumatic life events. They see five key forms of growth: improved relations with others, the identification of new possibilities for one's life, increased personal strength, spiritual change and enhanced appreciation of life. They believe that adversity may also provide opportunities for the development of important character traits, and character building in areas such as diligence, generosity, love, purpose and humility.

Most of us have resilience, but for many people it remains an untried strength. A traumatic event can force us to use our resilience, to take stock of our life, quantify the change that has occurred and then to do something about it — instead of drifting along as so often happens in an unprovoked life.

From the forge of terrible events, strong people can emerge and there is believed to be a correlation between the strength of events and the increase in personal strengths. It's thought that the key factor is self-discipline; when things go wrong and we fight back, we call upon our reserves of self-discipline and this in turn creates a feeling of accomplishment.

Modern medicine was responsible for my survival but determination, hard work, self-discipline and, of course, extraordinary support from family and friends has guided my recovery. After her stroke and before subsequent surgery, Jill Bolte Taylor walked and walked until, on the day prior to surgery she climbed the hill near her house and looked down over Boston, knowing that her determination to have a fit body would help her chances after surgery. She feared surgery might leave her without speech, but was similarly determined that she would try again if that happened.

The other person I've quoted in this book, Christine

Durham, has gone on to have a highly successful post-accident career, which she embarked on as soon as she could, determined to return to teaching when all evidence pointed to the contrary.

I intend to follow their example. Really, there's no choice. Cave in or get cracking.

Looking back — and forward

When I think back over these years, it's hard not to become an instant advocate for the rights of the disabled. If the news reports are right, and we are in for a tsunami of stroke patients (and other brain related illnesses that arise from an ageing population) then it seems to me that we have much to do. As governments struggle to get the funding formulae right — and we learn ever more about brain plasticity — we must ensure that rehab units are focused on care and rehabilitation, no matter what the reason for the patient coming in. Carer packages will be an important part of helping people to live independently.

But what about the myriad of small problems that plague the lives of people who are temporarily or permanently disabled? I'm talking of toilets, taxis, doorways, access to theatres and restaurants. These all need to be addressed. I have a friend who always ducked into a disabled toilet on the basis that they were more likely to be clean, empty and she'd only be there for a minute. After taking me out for a day, she no longer does it! It's that imaginative leap, putting yourself in the place of the person who needs that facility and doesn't have the choices of an able-bodied person.

The role of carers becomes critical. Who would ever have thought that at age 65 I would need personal carers to help me live independently in my own home? Their work is poorly paid, but vital. They must be people who really understand how important they are for those they care for, and not see their remuneration as an indicator of their value. Without them, nursing homes would be overflowing and people like me would be forced back into 'the system.' As the population ages, so will demand for good carers. I hope that my words can help others plan for that avalanche.

I manage my own package, which means I have been able to try carers out for their suitability for my needs. I now have a great team of women assisting me. I am so grateful for the professionalism and good humour they bring to my needs every single day. A good relationship with your carer has been shown to improve recovery; the benefits are long-term as well as daily companionship.

I intend getting back to the work of my pre-stroke life. Lucinda would have expected no less. When I look back, I can see that I have reinvented my professional life at least once a decade, and that each of these reinventions has coincided with a move of home. I've decided to keep that synchronicity going and so, in 2017, I'm moving home. I will leave Petrina and Gordon's back garden unit, which has been such an important part of my recovery, for an inner city suburb of Melbourne that I have loved since my university days.

The move will allow me to gently leave this part of my life behind and enter a future where I can commit to a life of meaning and purpose beyond that of my own needs. I have been the recipient of so much kindness and strength from others, and I have learnt so much, that it is now time for me to give back, to return fully to the world. To truly Stand Up!

Postscript

This book is about stroke and not cancer. However if I did not mention Lucinda's cancer and her death on May 5, 2015, I would be omitting a huge part of this story.

I have dedicated this book to her memory and I am dedicating my physiotherapy to her memory as she would want me to regain my previous mobility. I still have so much to live for — Emma and my grandchildren, my extended family and all my friends who are supporting me, AND keeping Lucinda's memory alive. I talk to her constantly. My love for her keeps growing.

Lucinda did not want to be identified by her cancer. We had a wonderful ceremony to celebrate her life with candles to signify the light of her soul. Indeed her name means light or illumination.

Her death led, naturally, to an unimaginably terrifying grief, a grief that eclipsed anything I had ever experienced. At first I just wanted to die with her. In these extreme moments, I was helped by a wonderful exercise that I had used in my work called 'saying hello again.' Michael White, a renowned narrative psychologist, developed this exercise. Sadly, he too died recently. The essence is to remember what you meant to the person you have lost, be it through death, divorce or any other aspect of profound loss. You then decide how you are going to BE to honour their memory of you.

I knew that Lucinda loved my courage and tenacity. I knew she loved my strong sense of family and my love for family and friends. I talk to her beautiful photo and feel her answers, as I tell her I am going off to physiotherapy to honour her memory. But I know her reply would have been, 'No Mum, you are going for YOU, so you gain as much independence as possible.' And she would have been right.

As I walk around my little house, I say 'See, I am working hard.' She just smiles with love. 'Get back to being a loving supportive mother and grandmother,' I hear her say. 'Go and enjoy your life as you always have.'

I was grateful to have tapped into the need for *meaning and purpose in life* during my rehabilitation, as I needed this focus to keep me going when Lucinda died. I don't mean finding meaning in her being taken so young. That remains cruelly incomprehensible. I mean finding the will to keep going myself. I know I am indeed blessed to be her mother, to have given life to that beautiful soul. My meaning and purpose in life now is to keep her memory alive in the hearts of all who love her. I have photos, candles and flowers everywhere. I am writing about her life and adding parts as people tell me their recollections and happy memories.

Naturally, there have been times when my will to tap into my strengths, essence and positive approach have been tested to the extreme. I needed to find a *sense of purpose* in what happened, in the terrible spread of Lucinda's cancer. As it grew, so did my devastation. Had I not suffered a stroke, how much more I could have done to help her. It would not have eased the grief, which I felt more about her illness than I had felt about my stroke. How could I not when my funny, kind, intelligent, giving girl was going through hell? I knew that to cope, I needed to find a sense of purpose. Throughout her illness, I sent flowers regularly and made soup and we talked on the phone and texted. I told her repeatedly of my great love for her. My purpose became one of expressing my love for her. Nothing else mattered.

It seemed important to help find ways for her wonderful work to continue. Richard decided that rather than flowers for her life celebration, we would ask people to donate to Melbourne's McAuley Women's Refuge. It has been my mission to see this fund grow. A program in Lucinda's name has been established to help children who have escaped family violence and similar situations to develop resilience.

Deakin University has announced the Dr Lucinda Jordan Research Award, an annual memorial award in recognition of Lucinda's work as a Research Fellow in the Deakin Law School and her passionate belief in the value of well articulated, quality research to inform and effect social change. The award will specifically promote those attributes that Lucinda was recognised for: collegiality, quality research and encouragement of early career researchers.

The fourth anniversary of my stroke was unimaginable. Lucinda was no longer there to share the date with me. I have found some peace in knowing that there is meaning in my life, in keeping her memory alive. Her friends, Nicki, Sarah and Bridget, visit me with their lovely children and when I see that their need to keep in touch is as great as mine, I am reminded how much Lucinda was loved and admired.

Lucinda would have fiercely wanted me to keep going and keep counting my prouds, so I do. I am proud to have lovely weekends with Emma and her family, where I have been able to walk around the house (Asher is excited to see me walking so well), play games with my grandchildren and enjoy the countryside. I am now using a normal walking stick, rather than the cumbersome four prong stick, and I can manage 50 metres from my house.

The real world is no longer out of bounds. I have enjoyed opera and ballet visits and recently I was thrilled to attend the 80th birthday celebration for Professor Graeme Clark. It was wonderful to be back in my professional world and celebrating the life of a remarkable man. As my colleagues from the Bionic Ear Institute, now the Bionics Institute, came over to talk to me, the difficult four years seemed to recede into the past.

I have started Transcendental Meditation and am loving practising it twice daily. This book has found a publisher and knowing that I will soon be contributing to others through my story has given me a definite purpose in life, as I start the fifth year after the stroke.

Petrina and Gordon have made a garden down the side of the house along the path that leads to my little house. We have planted Lucinda's favourite jasmine and gardenias. Family and friends are contributing to the garden with plants such as peony roses and bulbs. We want it be a fragrant garden in memory of a beautiful soul. Her legacy and memory will live on as her beautiful soul lives in our hearts and memories. I think back constantly to the wonderful heart of that little girl who would always ask, a hundred times on family birthdays, 'Are you happy?' Make no mistake. I remain heartbroken and devastated.

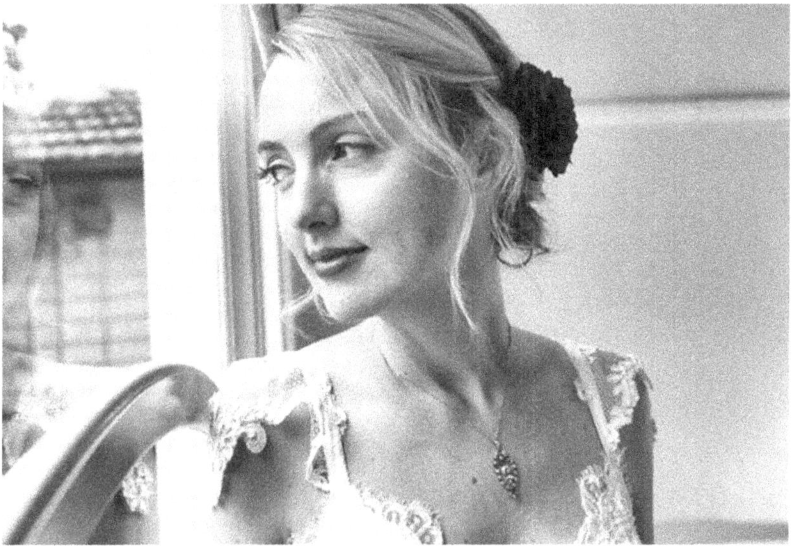

Epilogue

As I write this four and a half years after my stroke, I think, what have I learnt that will help you, the reader?

I encourage you to *maintain hope for your future*. Others will have their 'reasons' for suggesting that you need to be 'realistic' about your chances. But you must set your own expectations and create a course for your future.

Being true to oneself is critical. Encourage others to come on board with your hopes, dreams and expectations. Surround yourself with positivity and strength.

Above all else *nurture your relationships right now.* You just never know when the love you share with others will become your lifeline.

Be kind to others and, especially, compassionate with yourself. It's not possible, or human, to be relentlessly full of hope. There are good days and not-so good days. On the not-so good days, be as kind to yourself as you would be to another, and know that it will pass.

Believe in yourself and the possibility that you can create change. I knew that noise was detrimental to my wellbeing and rehabilitation. I kept requesting a solution. Now some years later, voices like mine have been heard and something has been done about noise levels in the rehab unit.

The importance of communication. This is really a comment for the entire health sector. It would have made such a difference to my daughters and sisters at various stages to have been consulted and heard. The minutes you spend explaining the situation to your patients and their families are as valuable as those you spend on the preservation of health. I would add that there were also times that I would have liked to have been given the courtesy of being seen as an intelligent person with something to offer the system.

Knowing oneself. I am fortunate to have had many opportunities to learn about myself. Often when coaching others, the light bulb has gone on and I have had an Aha! moment. Having said that, most of us know who we are and what is important to us. If you're not sure, find out. It will guide you and by staying true to that understanding I hope you will thrive. You may find, as others have done, that what you have learnt as a result of your stroke can direct you towards a new life, one even more in tune with your true self.

Keep it simple. Small, simple goals build up. It's like that old saying that the conquest of a mountain starts with one step. Then another… As the quote from St Francis of Assisi tells us, first do what is necessary, then what is possible and soon you will be doing the impossible.

I wish you, my reader, health, love and happiness.

Kathleen

Appendix

Personal strengths

(Taken largely from the work of Martin Seligman et al in 'authentic happiness')

Curiosity and interest in the world
Love of learning
Open
Wisdom
Perspective
Courage and bravery
Persistence
Integrity
Vitality
Adventurous
Love
Kindness
Calm
Being present
Compassion
Empathy
Social intelligence
Fairness and justice
Citizenship
Leadership
Loyalty

Teamwork
Forgiveness and mercy
Self control
Humility
Modesty
Prudence
Appreciation of beauty and excellence
Gratitude
Hope, optimism, future mindedness
Humour and playfulness
Spirituality, faith and purpose

Acknowledgements

I am eternally grateful to my daughters, Emma and Lucinda. They were my constant rocks through those first terrifying weeks and months. Emma would pack up and leave her family in Western Victoria to be with me and Lucinda at the weekends. I am grateful to my son-in-law, Piet, for holding the fort so that Emma could be with me. Also to my grandchildren, Asher, Rose and Jack for sparing their darling Mum for days at a time.

The reader will have noticed that the bond between me and Emma and Lucinda was pivotal to this story.

Lucinda was extraordinary. She was constantly by my bedside. Her presence comforted me greatly. Despite being encouraged by others to close down the structure around my business, she resisted. Instead, knowing how important my company iNTUITIVE iNSIGHTS was to me, she threw herself with her usual commitment and intelligence into keeping it going for me.

I am grateful to my son-in-law Richard. His was a loving presence and he offered lots of practical help as well. He supported Lucinda so that she could be with me. They started and managed the visitors' roster and Richard downloaded beautiful music onto my iPod to calm me.

My darling sister Petrina was an amazing advocate for me in those first two years, and then a compassionate support through Lucinda's illness and death. I am so grateful. Not only did she welcome me into her home, she remained vigilant to my emotional needs and cheered me on with every step in my progress. I would not have reached the independence I have without her. I am indeed blessed.

In a way, this book is about the love and support of family. I am grateful to my four sisters and my four brothers-in-law. Without them all I would not have recovered as well as I have. Indeed I might not be living at home again. And to my nieces and nephews, for their love and concern, humour and support.

Friends and colleagues on the board of the Bionic Institute, whose concern and support lifted my spirits and helped me to understand that I had a professional life to return to.

My wonderful friends have also been instrumental in my progress towards my old life. Liz, my dearest friend of more than 40 years, was a treasure. We continued to share laughter when she visited me. She was determined to have me back sharing the fun times we always used to enjoy. In time, we enjoyed going out for meals. Even going for medical appointments with her was fun and felt normal. At last came the day we went to the ballet again. We were not seated in our usual seats of 20 years in the stalls on opening nights. We were in special wheelchair accessible seats right up in the roof. We went for Saturday matinees. My fatigue pushed evening outings into the future. At least I was there! And Liz made it fun pretending we were in the Royal box.

My dearest friend in England, Diana and her daughter, Helen, my goddaughter, were with me constantly in spirit. They sent letters, emails, cards, texts and flowers. Until they could get to visit me, they rang and reminded me constantly from afar of how loved I am.

I also thank:

Jen and Alice for fun visits and, once I was up to it, for outings into the *real world* to galleries and restaurants.

Darling Marilyn for regular visits, delicious homemade cake and outings, and Bosco too, when you were able to join us. Marilyn took me to the cinema and the theatre and to their home for wonderful lunches. I am so very grateful.

Judith for taking me to the all-important appointments at the day spa.

Ann and David for happy visits and outings and for reminding me I still have a professional life to get back to.

Trischa for taking the burden of running my financial life from Lucinda and for happy visits and yummy soup. Her husband Don for delicious homemade biscuits.

Berenice for calling in on her way home from work to give me neck massages whilst I was in rehab. Then once I was home, for happy visits over delicious lunches and for keeping in touch through thick and thin.

Gael, my masseuse of nearly 20 years, for coming to rehab and home to give me wonderful remedial massages.

Rosie and Dick for our bridge games in rehab and their home. Rosie, for taking me to the hairdresser and medical appointments.

My friend Cassandra for your professional counsel. Your willingness to talk to my family, your neurological expertise and knowledge of the geriatric system, alleviated their concerns in those first confusing and distressing months, and your visits to me were very reassuring. We are all grateful.

Jenny, Sally, David and Moya for visits, outings and phone calls and the constant reminder that friendships endure a lifetime. Margaret, a lifelong friend, for lending me your stunning apartment at Docklands so I could escape rehab with Helen and Diana for Lucinda's wedding.

Many friends brought wonderful picnics, which we shared under the trees. In particular I thank Megan, Trent and Paula for delicious goodies as an escape from rehab, then also at home. Paula, my favourite cousin, I thank you for coming all the way from Perth on a number of important occasions.

My Beliefs Team, you were all pivotal to my progress. Pam, Kate, Liz and Vicki, I acknowledge with gratitude your ongoing support. You were my cheerleaders.

Kate for every time she came to Melbourne with her wonderful smile and positive wisdom. Kate would walk in and my worries would evaporate. We also had lots of phone calls. These helped me focus on the positives.

There are so many people who helped me recover.

I acknowledge with gratitude, my neurosurgeon Michael Wong. His expertise gave me a chance at life. His medical team and the nurses at RMH. The Allied Health professionals, physiotherapists, occupational therapists and speech therapists who all worked enthusiastically with me, matching my determination to get well.

My counsellors, Pam and Franca. Their belief in me gave me strength and helped me to overcome the emotional barriers to progress. My psychiatrist Brett Coulson, who helped me through the frightening psychotic phase. My GP, Suzanne Hoggarth, for her constant care.

A special acknowledgement to many of my clients. Bernadette in Bahrain, Trish and John in Canberra, and Cecilia in New Zealand. Your belief in me and your support encouraged me. In particular, I thank Michelle McLean, CEO at Cornwall Stodart lawyers, for all the support she and her firm have provided.

Danny, thank you for modelling the benefits of meditation. Brian, thank you (as always) for your ongoing support and friendship and, in particular, thank you for introducing me to Faye and Transcendental Meditation. Faye, for your inspirational instruction in TM.

Peter and Paul Apostolis for their wonderful mCareWatch. Knowing that I can muster help at the press of a button has given me the security to push my boundaries at home without fear of the consequences of a fall.

I acknowledge the Transitional Care team led by Catherine, who helped me make the huge move from institutional living to being at home again. I am grateful to Emelia, the OT who secured this service for me, as well as her gentle encouragement throughout my time in slow stream rehab.

At the time of writing, I have ongoing physiotherapy with Kim and Kathy. Their expertise as neuro-physiotherapists and their Bobath training is making an incredible difference to my progress. My OTs Tim, Natalie and Carly are helping with the functional challenges of living independently.

I acknowledge the federal government for the EACH package that makes it financially possible for me to be living at home. I am fortunate to have Baptcare Independence at Home, BIAH.

Thank you to case manager Bernadette who oversees my care and the management of my package and provides a wonderful team of carers who have made living at home possible. I thank each of them for their dedication and contribution, with special thanks to Angela and Lesley.

I am deeply grateful to my sister Petrina and her husband

Gordon and their children Lara, Daniel and Genevieve for making me so welcome and feeling loved in my home in their garden. Also to Shep for pointing out hundreds of times a day that life is about chasing sticks.

I am blessed to be surrounded by a wonderful community of neighbours, Ruth, Helen, Margaret, Helen and John. Thank you for coffee catch-ups, drinks, festive meals, help into taxis. The support of knowing you are all around gives me a great sense of comfort and belonging.

The publication of the book has involved many people. Special thanks to Margot for your photographs, Liz for your creative design advice, Gordon for publishing advice and Jasmine and her team at Impact Press for making it happen.

To Neil, thank you for your friendship and for identifying the opportunity to connect me with Vicki. Synchrodestiny in action! Thank you also for your marketing advice to get *Standing Up!* out there.

Finally my co-author, Victoria Steggall. Vicki, this book would have remained an elusive dream without you. I am grateful that my belief that *Standing Up!* will inspire others is that bit closer to reality. Your professionalism, expertise and friendship have made this project joyful.

Kathleen Jordan
iNTUITIVE iNSIGHTS

Bibliography

Bauby, J	*The Diving Bell & the Butterfly,* Fourth Estate, Great Britain 1997
Bolte Taylor, J	*My Stroke of Insight, A Brain Scientist's Personal Journey,* Penguin US 2008
Boniwell, I	*Positive Psychology in a Nutshell, The science of happiness,* Open University Press 2012
Cahalan, Susannah	*Brain on Fire, My month of madness.* Particular Books, Penguin 2012
Durham, C	*Doing up Buttons,* Penguin Group Australia 1997 (now published as *Unlocking my Brain,* Ventura Press 2014)
Frankel, V	*Man's Search for Meaning,* originally published in German in 1946, this edition published by Rider, Random House, UK 2008
Hefferon,K	*Positive Psychology and the Body, The Somatopsychic Side to Flourishing,* Open University Press 2013
HeartMath	I encourage readers to explore the HeartMath website. www.heartmath.com

Joseph, S	*What Doesn't Kill Us, The new psychology of post traumatic growth,* Piatkus Great Britain 2012
Linley Alex P and Stephen Joseph (eds)	*Positive Psychology in Practice,* John Wiley and Sons, New Jersey 2004
Peterson, C	*A Primer in Positive Psychology,* Oxford University Press, NY 2004
Seligman, M	*Authentic Happiness,* Simon & Schuster Inc 2002, republished by William Heinemann 2011
Seligman, M and Peterson, C	*Character Strengths and Virtues, A handbook and classification* Oxford University Press 2004
Seligman, M	*Flourish: A Visionary New Understanding of Happiness and Well-being,* William Heinemann, Australia 2011
St Luke's Innovative Resources	www.innovativeresources.org

www.ingramcontent.com/pod-product-compliance
Lightning Source LLC
Chambersburg PA
CBHW031154270326
41931CB00006B/262
* 9 7 8 0 6 4 8 4 6 0 4 4 2 *